# Baby Names

*The Baby Name Bible – The Most Popular Baby Names of 2018! Includes Baby Names for Boys and Girls as well as the Latest Trends!*

*(Contains 2 Manuscripts: Baby Names & The Essential Guide to Raising a Healthy Baby)*

## Jessica Ford

# Baby Names

*The Ultimate Book of Baby Names –
Includes the Latest Trends, Meanings,
Origins and Spiritual Significance*

The following eBook is reproduced below with the goal of providing information that is as accurate and as reliable as possible. Regardless, purchasing this eBook can be seen as consent to the fact that both the publisher and the author of this book are in no way experts on the topics discussed within, and that any recommendations or suggestions made herein are for entertainment purposes only. Professionals should be consulted as needed before undertaking any of the action endorsed herein.

This declaration is deemed fair and valid by both the American Bar Association and the Committee of Publishers Association and is legally binding throughout the United States.

Furthermore, the transmission, duplication or reproduction of any of the following work, including precise information, will be considered an illegal act, irrespective whether it is done electronically or in print. The legality extends to creating a secondary or tertiary copy of the work or a recorded copy and is only allowed with an express written consent of the Publisher. All additional rights are reserved.

The information in the following pages is broadly considered to be a truthful and accurate account of facts, and as such any inattention, use or misuse of the information in question by the reader will render any resulting actions solely under their purview.

There are no scenarios in which the publisher or the original author of this work can be in any fashion deemed liable for any hardship or damages that may befall them after undertaking information described herein.

Additionally, the information found on the following pages is intended for informational purposes only and should thus be considered, universal. As befitting its nature, the information presented is without assurance regarding its continued validity or interim quality. Trademarks that are mentioned are done without written consent and can in no way be considered an endorsement from the trademark holder.

# Table of Contents

# Introduction

Congratulations on downloading your personal copy of *Baby Names: The Ultimate Book of Baby Names – Includes the Latest Trends, Meanings, Origins and Spiritual Significance.* Thank you for doing so.

The following chapters will provide you with lots of different baby names from around the world. Each chapter is broken down into boy, girl, and unisex names. Every name has information about what it means and where it originated along with many other interesting facts.

Picking your child's name is the first hardest decision you will have to make in your child's life, so why not have a little bit of help. This book has lots of names, and you are sure to find one that is perfect for your baby.

There are plenty of books on this subject on the market, thanks again for choosing this one! Every effort was made to ensure it is full of as much useful information as possible. Please enjoy!

# Trending

## Boys

**Liam**: The number one trending boy name is German. The Irish derivative of the German name *William* that contains the elements *wil* meaning 'desire' and *helm* meaning 'helmet' and together means 'strong-willed warrior'.

**Noah**: The number two trending boy name is of Hebrew origin and means 'comfort' or 'rest'. In the Old Testament, Noah built the Ark and saved his family and the animals from the Great Flood. He got a sign from God in the form of the rainbow. He fathered three sons Japheth, Ham, and Shem.

**Elijah**: The number three trending boy name is of Hebrew origin and means 'My God is Yahweh'. In the Old Testament, Elijah was a miracle worker and prophet. Elijah confronted King Ahab and Queen Jezebel over their worship of the idol Ba'al. He did not die but was carried to heaven in a chariot of fire. Since Elijah was popular in medieval tales, and the name was given by many saints, the name was regularly used during the middle ages. During medieval England, the name was spelled, *Elis*.

**Logan**: The fourth trending boy name is of Celtic origin. It was from the surname *Lagan* that was derived from a Scottish place name that means 'little hollow'.

**Mason**: The fifth trending boy name is of French origin. It is from the surname that is given to stone workers.

**James**: The sixth trending boy name is of Hebrew origin, and it means 'follower'. There were three James mentioned in the New Testament. *Saint James the Greater* was beheaded under Herod Agrippa. *James the Lesser* was the son of Alphaeus. *James the Just* was the brother of Jesus. The name has been used in England since the 1400s. It is more common in Scotland since it has seen several kings named James.

**Aiden**: The seventh trending boy name is of Celtic origin and means 'little fire'. It is an anglicized form of *Aodhan*. In the last part of the 1900s, it has risen in popularity in the US because of the sound *aden*.

**Ethan**: The eighth trending boy name is of Hebrew origin meaning 'firm', 'enduring', 'solid', or 'strong'. In the Old Testament, there weren't many characters with this name; the most notable is *Ethan the Ezrahite*. He was the writer of Psalm 89. It was used after the Protestant Reformation in the English-speaking world. It got popular in America because of *Ethan Allen (1738-1789)*.

**Lucas**: The ninth trending boy name is of Latin origin and means 'light'. It is a variation of the Biblical name Luke. It is an English form of a Greek name meaning from Lucania. In the Bible, Luke was a physician that traveled with the Apostle Paul. He is thought to have been of Greek descent.

**Michael**: The tenth trending boy name is of Hebrew origin that means who is like God? Michael was one of the seven archangels. In the Old Testament in the book of Daniel, he is named as the protector of Israel. In Revelation, he is portrayed as heaven's army's leader. He is considered the patron saint of soldiers.

**William**: The next trending boy name is of German origin. It is derived from the elements *wil* meaning 'desire' or will and *helm* meaning 'protection' or 'helmet'. It is a variation of the name *Willahelm*.

**Sebastian**: The next trending boy name is of Latin origin. It is a version of the name *Sebastianus* which means 'from *Sebaste'*. This is a town in Asia Minor. Its name comes from the Greek *sebastos* meaning 'venerable'. Saint Sebastian was a Roman soldier that was martyred. When it was discovered he was a Christian, he was tied and shot with arrows. This didn't kill him.

**Joseph**: The next trending boy name is of Hebrew origin. It is from the Greek word *Ioseph* which is from the Hebrew name *Yosef* which means 'he will add'. In the Old Testament Joseph is a son of Jacob and husband to Rachel. He was his father's favorite and his brothers sold him into slavery. While in Egypt, Joseph gained fame and became an advisor to the pharaoh.

**David**: The next trending boy name is of Hebrew origin. It is derived from *Dawid* that was derived from *dwd* meaning 'beloved'. David was one of the greatest kings of Israel and ruled in the 900s BC. The most famous story is when he defeated Goliath, a huge Philistine. Jesus is said to be a descendant of him.

**Gabriel**: The next trending boy name is of Hebrew origin. It is derived from the Hebrew *Gavri'el*, meaning 'God is my strong man'. It could also be derived from *ever* which means 'hero or strong man'. Gabriel is an archangel and appears as God's messenger. In the Old Testament, he was sent to help Daniel interpret dreams. In the New Testament, he was sent to announce the birth of John and Jesus.

## Girls

**Emma**: The number one trending girl name is of Latin origin. It was originally short for any Germanic name that began with the element *ermen* that means 'universal or whole'. Emma of Normandy was the wife of King Ethelred II and King Canute. She introduced the name to England. It also is derived by an Austrian saint that was called *Hemma*.

**Olivia**: The second trending girl name was popularized by Shakespeare. It was spelled this way by William Shakespeare in the comedy, Twelfth Night. Olivia is a wealthy, pampered Countess. In ancient Greece, this name meant 'olive' and was symbolic for Athena. It was also a token of fertility and peace. Olive wreaths were given as awards at the Olympic Games.

**Ava**: The third most trending name is from different origins. It has roots in German, Persian, and English.

This name originally was a short form of German names that began with the element *avi* that probably meant 'desired'. In Persia, the name means 'sound or voice'. In the English origin, it is a variation of Eve.

**Isabella**: The fourth trending name of Hebrew origin. It is the Latin form of Isabel. It is a variation of Elizabeth that means 'devoted to God'. This name was held by many medieval royals like queen consorts of Hungary, Holy Roman Empire, Portugal, France, and England. And the powerful Queen Isabella of Castile.

**Sophia**: The fifth trending name is of Greek origin and means wisdom. This name comes from an early possibly mythical saint that died from grief after her daughters were slain during Emperor Hadrian's reign. Legends arose due to the misunderstanding of the phrase *Hagia Sophia,* meaning 'Holy Wisdom'. This is the name of the basilica in Constantinople. This name was common with royalty during the Middle Ages and became popular in Britain by the German Hanover House when they gained control of the throne in the 1900s.

**Mia**: The sixth trending name has German, Dutch, and Scandinavian roots. It is a derivative of Maria. It matches with the Italian word *mia* that means 'mine'. It is the Israeli abbreviation of *Michal.* In Latin, it means 'wished for child, bitter, or rebellion'.

**Charlotte**: The seventh trending name is of French origin, and it means 'free'. It is the feminine form of Charles and shares nicknames of Charley or Charlie.

Other nicknames are Char, Lotta, and Lottie. Carlotta is the Italian form of Charlotte.

**Amelia**: The eighth trending name is of Hebrew origin. The Germanic spelling *Amalia* means 'work'. It could also be a variant of *Emilia* meaning 'rival'. In Latin, it means 'striving and industrious'. The Teutonic meaning is 'defender'.

**Abigail**: The ninth trending name is of Hebrew origin *Avigayil* meaning 'my father is joy'. When used as an English name, Abigail became common after the Protestant Reformation. It was popular with the Puritans, too. In the Old Testament, Abigail was Nabal's wife. After he died, she became King David's third wife. Abigail called herself a servant. In the 1600s the name was slang for servant. The name was not fashionable after that but was revived in the 1900s.

**Emily**: The tenth trending name is of Latin origin and means 'eager or striving'. It is an English cognate of the Latin name *Aemilia*, which derives from *Aemilius* that is an Old Roman family name that is derived from *Aemulus* meaning 'trying to equal or excel, rival'. The name Emily means 'strong, pretty, simple, classic, and feminine'.

**Camila**: The next trending girl name is of Portuguese and Spanish origin. It is a variation of *Camilla*. *Camilla* is the feminine of *Camillus*. This name is a legendary warrior maiden of the Volsci. *Camillus* goes back to Ancient Roman and its meaning is unknown. It may have been related to Latin *camillus* meaning 'a youth employed in religious services'.

**Ella**: The next trending girl name is of French origin. It's a form of the name *Alienor*. She was called *Aenor* by her mother and was called *Alia Aenor* which means 'the other Aenor' by the Occitan. It is also short for *Eleanor*.

**Zoey**: The next trending girl name is of Greek, Italian, and English origins. It means 'life' in Greek. It was adopted by Jews as a translation of Eve. Zoe has been used since the 1800s. It is more common with Christians and has many different spellings.

**Penelope**: The next trending girl name is of English and Greek mythology origins. It is derived from the Greek *penelops,* a type of duck. It also has the elements of *pene* meaning 'weft or threads' and *ops* meaning 'eye or face'. It was the name of Odysseus's wife in Homer's epic poem 'Odyssey'.

**Mila**: The next trending girl name is of Slavic origin. It has the elements *milu* meaning 'dear and gracious.' In Slavic, it means 'hard working or industrious'. In Russia, it means 'dear one'. It is a pet form of the names Miloslava, Camila, Ludmila, Milica, Milan, and Milena. It has been connected to the Spanish name *Milagros* that means 'miracles'.

# Unisex

**Addison**: This unisex name is of Hebrew origin and began life as an English surname, which means 'son of Adam'. It is also a Scottish patronymic surname that 'means son of Addie'. In the Scottish Lowlands, it is a nickname for Adam.

**Ash**: This unisex name is of Hebrew origin and began life as an English place-name. The Hebrew meaning is 'happy'. The English meaning is 'ash tree'. This name was derived from the element *Æsc* meaning 'ash tree' and *tun* which means 'enclosure, village, settlement, or town'.

**Aubrey**: This unisex name has roots in France and means 'ruler of elves or supernatural being'. It is an English given name. It is a Norman French version of the German given name *Alberic*. The name was derived from the element *alf or elf* and *ric* which means 'power'.

**Bailey**: This unisex name has roots in Middle English that referred to someone in the position of steward or official, bailiff, warrant officer. It is a topographical name for a person who resided near the outer wall of a castle. The name was derived from the Old English, *beg,* meaning 'berry' plus *leah* meaning 'woodland clearing'.

**Bobbie**: This unisex name is of German origin and means 'shining, bright, famed'. This name was introduced to the English by the Normans. In England, it is slang for policeman. Short for Robert which is derived from Old German *Hrodebert* with the elements *hruod* meaning 'fame' and *behrt* meaning 'bright'.

**Brett**: This unisex name is from the Celtic origin meaning 'a Breton'. In the English origin, it means a native of Brittany.

**Brook**: This unisex name has mixed origins of Old English and Old German. It means 'small stream'.

**Charlie**: This unisex name has English, French, and Germanic origins. It comes from the Old English *ceorl* that means 'man'. In French and German meanings, it stands for 'free man'.

**Corey**: This unisex name has been borrowed from the Irish. It has several origins. It originated from a Gaelic surname *coire* that means a 'hollow, a seething pool, or a cauldron' and is said to be a dweller near or in a hollow. In German and English, the name means 'God's peace'. It also holds origins with the Norse name of *Kori*.

**Dakota**: This unisex name is of Native American origin and means 'ally or friend' in the Santee and Yankton-Yanktonai dialects of the Lakota Sioux tribe from the northern Mississippi valley.

**Daryl**: This unisex name has origins in Old French and Middle English. In French, it is a place name that means 'open'. In English, it means 'dearly loved, and darling'. This name dates back to the 1200s as both a given and surname in France.

**Eli**: This unisex name is of Hebrew origin and means 'high, elevated, or my God'. Eli was a judge and priest in the Old Testament that raised Samuel who became a prophet. Within the Greek origin, it means 'defender of man'.

**Frankie**: This unisex name has many different origins. In German, it means 'javelin'. In Latin, it means 'free'. In English, it means 'honest'. Frankie is mostly used as a nickname for Frances, Francine, Francesco, or Frank.

**Gray**: This unisex name is of English origin. It was used as a nickname for anyone that had gray beards or hair. In Ireland and Scotland, it has been translated from different Gaelic surnames that were derived from *riabhach* meaning 'gray or brindled'.

**Harper**: This unisex name is of Scottish origin. It originated in the Dalriadan region of Scotland and is part of the Buchanan Clan. Harper was Anglicization of the German name *Harpfer*, meaning to 'play the harp'.

**Hayden**: This unisex name has many origins. It was an English surname that was derived from different place names. It is derived from the elements *heg* meaning 'hay and *denu* 'valley'; *heg* meaning 'hay' and *dun* meaning 'hill'; *hege* meaning 'hedge' and *dun* meaning 'hill'. It also has Welsh origins from the Hayden meaning 'fire' that was derived from the Celtic name *Aidan*.

**Jamie**: This unisex name has many origins. It has roots in Hebrew, Scottish, and English. They all mean 'supplanter or seized by the heel'. It is the feminine form or James. There are many different spellings of this name: Jamie, Jaime, and Jamey.

**Jesse**: This unisex name is of Hebrew origin from the name *Yishai, which* means 'gift'. Jesse is from the Old Testament. He was the father of David. The stem of Jesse is used to describe David's family. Jesse was a wealthy man who held a high position in Bethlehem. Different spellings of this name are Jessie, Jessee or shortened to Jess.

**Kennedy**: This unisex name is of Gaelic origin and means 'helmeted leader or armored head'. The name is derived from two elements *ceann* meaning 'head' and *eidigh* meaning 'ugly' or *ceann* meaning 'head' and *eide* meaning 'armor' so the name could mean 'helmet headed'.

**Morgan**: This unisex name comes from Scotland, Brittany, and Wales. The male version *Morcant* is derived from *mor* meaning 'sea' and *cant* meaning 'circle' that means 'sea chief or sea defender'.

**Peyton**: This unisex name is of English origin and was a place name, meaning 'Paega's town'. It was originally a surname in Sussex. It is a version of Payton.

**River**: This unisex name is of English origin and means 'river or large creek'. It also has Shakespearean origins. Lord Rivers is Lady Grey's brother in King

Henry the Sixth III, and Earl Rivers is King Edward's Queen's brother in King Richard III.

**Rudy**: This unisex name is of German origin. It is short for Rudolf or Rudiger. Rudiger comes from the Old German *Hruodiger* meaning 'spear fame' or 'fame with a spear'. The name derives from the elements *hroud* meaning 'fame' and *ger* meaning 'spear'. Rudolf means 'famed wolf'.

**Stevie**: This unisex name is of Greek origin and means 'victorious or crown'. It has been used as a shortened form of Stephanie or Stephen.

**Tanner**: This unisex name is of English origin. It was a surname that referred to an occupational name. The Old English word *tannere* signified a person who was a tanner of animal skins. They produced leather for everyday items like armor, saddles, horse harnesses, or shoes in medieval times and even before. This word was influenced by the Celtic word for oak tree. The tree bark was used in tanning. The surname was first spelled Tannur in the 1300s.

**Taylor**: This unisex name is of English origin. It is a surname and comes from the word *tailor*. It ultimately came from the Latin word *taliare* meaning 'to cut'.

**Tyler**: This unisex name is from English origin and means 'maker of tiles or bricks'. This surname was derived from the old French *tieuleor, tieulier* meaning 'tile maker or tiler' and the Middle English *tyler, tylere* meaning 'a tile or a brick'. The name was originally an occupational name for a brick or tile layer or maker.

**West**: This unisex name has both German and English origins. From the Middle English, Middle High German west, so it was a topographic name for a person that lived toward the west of a settlement. A regional name for people who migrated from the west.

**Winter**: This unisex name is of English origins and began as a surname that dates as far back as the ninth century. In Greek mythology, the seasons were placed to give Persephone's time between her lovers on Hades and Earth. Persephone was told to stay with Hades in the Winter until Spring. This name means the 'coldest season of the year'. The Native American meaning is 'bringing of renewal'.

# Celtic

## Boys

**Angus**: This boy name is an Anglicized form of the Gaelic *Aonghas*. This is derived from the elements of *one and choice*. A Scottish version is *Aonghus*. *Aonghus* means 'one strength'. This is derived from the elements *one* and *gus* meaning 'energy, strength, or force'. He was the Irish god of youth and love. The Irish form is *Aengus*.

**Bowden**: This boy name is of Angle-Saxon origin and is from two sources. It can be a place name meaning a 'dweller at the top of a hill' or from the Old English phrase, *befan dune* that means 'above the hill'. It could also be from any place called Bowdon or Bowden. There are places in Scotland from the Gaelic both *an duin* that translates to 'house on the hill'.

**Driscoll**: This boy name is of Irish origin. It is a reduced for of the Gaelic *O' hEidirsceoil* meaning 'descendant of the messenger', from *eidirsceol* meaning 'news bearer, intermediary, and go between'.

**Fergus:** This boy name is of Irish origin and means 'man of vigor'. It is derived from the elements *fear* meaning 'man' and *gus* meaning 'vigor'. This is a popular Irish or Scottish given name. It originally came from the Proto-Celtic elements *wiros* meaning 'man' and *gustus* meaning 'choice, force, or vigor'. The first reference is to a Pictish king. The surname of

Fergusson or Ferguson is normal across Scotland but more in Ayrshire and Perthshire. In Ireland, the Ferris family gets its surname from *O'Fearghusa*.

**Kegan**: This boy name is of Irish, Gaelic, and Celtic origin. They all mean 'fiery and small'.

**Maddox**: This boy name is of Welsh origin. It originally was a surname meaning son of Madoc. Madoc or Madog was a Welsh prince that supposedly sailed to the New World three hundred years before Columbus did. The name means 'fortunate' and is derived from the element *mad*.

**Owyn**: This boy name is of Irish, Welsh, and Celtic origins and means 'young fighter'. It is a variation of Owen.

**Sloane**: This boy name is of Irish origin. It was used as a surname but was Anglicized from the Irish *O'Sluaghain. Sluaghhadain* is a version of the ancient Gaelic name *Sluaghadh* that means 'raid'. Therefore, Sloane means 'little raider'.

**Tiernay**: This boy name is of Irish origin. It means 'chief or lord' and implies 'lord of the household'. It is the Anglicized form of the surname *Tighearnach*.

**Weylin**: This boy name is of Celtic origin and means 'son of the wolf'. It is a variation of Waylon.

## Girls

**Brygid**: This girl name is of Gaelic origin and means 'strength or exalted one'. It is a variation of the name, Bridget.

**Cordelia**: This girl name is of Celtic origin. It became famous as the heroine in Shakespeare's King Lear. The character was based on queen Cordelia. The meaning is uncertain but could be derived from the Latin *cor* meaning 'heart'. It is also linked with the Welsh name *Creiddylad* meaning 'jewel of the sea'. It could also come from the French *Coeur de lion* meaning 'heart of a lion'.

**Etain**: This girl name is of Irish origin and means 'jealousy'. The Irish myth holds Etain as a beautiful fairy who was turned into a scarlet fly by a jealous queen. She was blown off an ocean for several years. When she was able to come back to Ireland, she fell into some wine and was swallowed by a woman who wanted a child. Etain was reborn and married a King of Ireland.

**Fiona**: This girl name is of Gaelic origin and means 'fair or white'. Fiona is the most well-known in a group of Gaelic names. This is ironic since it is without genuine roots. It was first found in the *Ossianic* poem of James Macpherson. It became popular in the late 1800s as a feminine pen name for a Scottish writer.

**Gwyndolin**: This girl name is of Welsh origin and means 'white ring'. It is derived from the elements *gwen* meaning 'blessed, white, fair' and *dolen* meaning 'ring'. This is a mythical queen who fought her husband in battle and defeated him.

**Kaedence**: This girl name is of Celtic origin and means 'to march in rhythm'.

**Lyonesse**: This girl name is of Celtic origin and means 'little lion'.

**Morrigan**: This girl name is of Irish origin. It is derived from *Mor Rioghain* that means 'great queen'. In an Irish myth, she is a goddess of war and took the form of a cow.

**Oriana**: This girl name is of Latin origin meaning 'rising sun'. This medieval name is exotic and strong. She was the love of knight Amadis.

**Venetia**: This girl name is of Celtic origin. It is a place name the means 'blessed'. It is a form of Gwyneth.

## Unisex

**Arleigh**: This unisex name is of Old English origin. It is a variant of Arley and Harley. It made its way into popularity with the Scots and became one of the top Celtic names. It means 'vow or pledge'.

**Arlyss**: This unisex name is of Welsh origin meaning 'snowdrop'. It is a variation of Eirlys. This name is attractive and has a lot of flair and character.

**Bevan**: This unisex name is of Welsh, Gaelic, and Celtic origin. It is derived from *ab-evan* that means 'son of Evan'. The Gaelic meaning is 'fair lady'. The Celtic origin is 'youthful warrior'.

**Brennan**: This unisex name is of Gaelic and Irish origin. It comes from the surname Brennan which in Irish is spelled *o'Braonain* and means the 'descendant of Braonan'. The Gaelic personal name

*Braonan* comes from the Irish *braon* that means 'sorrow'. In other cases, the name may have come from the name, Brendan.

**Caradoc**: This unisex name is of Welsh origin and means 'amiable, affection'. In Celtic origin, it means 'dearly loved'. This ancient Celtic name is shared with a Knight of the Round Table and a Welsh King. This name was very common in the Middle Ages. This name appears in Welsh Triads as Arthur's chief elder and one of the knights of the Britain Island.

**Carrington**: This unisex name is of Celtic origin and is a surname and place name. It means 'town of the marsh'.

**Kerwin**: This unisex name is of Irish, Gaelic, and Celtic origin. It means 'small black one' in Irish, 'little black one' in Gaelic, and 'dark skinned' in Celtic.

**Makenna**: This unisex name is of Gaelic origin. It was originally a surname *Mac Cionaodha* that means 'son of Cionaodh'. It is a variation of McKenna and means 'happy one'.

**Sheridan**: This unisex name is an Irish surname that is derived from *O' Sirideain* that means 'descendant of *Siridean*'. The elements *O* meaning 'descendant of' and *Sirideain* is a nickname for 'elf'. It is possible since elves were known to be mischievous creatures, someone was given this nickname because they were somewhat mischievous as well. In Gaelic, the name *Siridean* means 'searcher'.

**Tiernan**: This unisex name is of Irish origin and means 'little lord'. It comes from an Old Gaelic name *MacTighearnain* that means 'son of Tierna'. This name means 'master or lord'. Variations of this surname are O'Tiernan, MacTiernan, McTiernan, and Tiernan.

# Nordic

## Boys

**Bard**: This boy name is of Norwegian origin. It is from the Old Norse *Bardr* that comes from the elements *badu,* meaning 'battle' and *fridr,* meaning 'peace'. Therefore, it means 'battle against peace'.

**Calder**: This boy name is of Old Norse origin via Scotland. It is a place name from any places like Cawdor, Caldor, or Calder. Calder in Thurso was recorded in the early 1200s with the spelling *Kalfadal* which is derived from the elements *kalfr* meaning 'calf' and *dalr* meaning 'valley'. From the Welsh origin, it is derived from the elements *caled* meaning 'hard or violent' and *dwfr* meaning 'stream or water'. So, its meaning could be 'valley of the calf' or 'violent water'.

**Eirik**: This boy name is of Norse origin and means 'eternal ruler' or 'forever strong'. This is a variation of Eric. It was once popular with Scandinavian royalty since many kings of Denmark, Norway, and Sweden used it.

**Gandalf**: This boy name is from Norse Mythology origin and means elf with a wand. It comes from the elements gandr, meaning cane, staff, or wand and alfr, meaning elf. The famous bearer of the name is the beloved character in the novel, *The Lord of the Rings* written by J.R.R. Tolkien.

**Ivar**: This boy name is of Danish, Norwegian, and Swedish origins. It is an Old Norse name *Ivarr*. It is derived from elements *yr* meaning 'bow or yew' and *arr* meaning 'warrior'. Therefore, it means 'warrior with a bow'. It was brought to England by the Scandinavian invaders during the Middle Ages. It was adopted by Wales, Scotland, and Ireland.

**Kensley**: This boy name has origins in both Old Norse and Gaelic meaning from a 'clearing with a spring'. It is derived from the elements *kelda* that means 'well or spring' and the Old English word meaning *leah* that means 'wood or clearing'. It is a place name showing the bearer comes from near a clearing with a spring.

**Odin**: This boy name is of Old Norse origin and means 'fury'. It is derived from the element *odr* that means 'inspiration or fury'. *Odin* was the god of death, wisdom, and war in Norse mythology.

**Stig**: This boy name has origins in Old Norse and Danish. It is a variation of *Stigr* and originates from the Old Norse meaning 'route'.

**Sven**: This boy name is of Old Norse origin and means boy. Sven is from Scandinavia of Old Norse origins. It derives from the element *sven* that means 'boy'.

**Viggo**: This boy name is of Old Norse origin and means battle. It is derived from the element *vig* meaning 'war or fight'.

# Girls

**Aslog**: This girl name is from Old Norse and Danish origins and means 'woman engaged to God'. It is a variation of the name *Aslaug*. It derives from the element *ass* meaning 'God' and *laug* meaning 'betrothed woman'.

**Astrid**: This girl name is of Old Norse origin and means 'divine beauty'. It is derived from the elements *ass* meaning 'God' and *fridr* meaning 'beloved or beautiful'. It's more popular with Scandinavian languages because of the creator of Pippi Longstocking's author Astrid Lindgren.

**Brenna**: This girl name is of Old Norse origin and means 'sword'. It is a variation of Brenda. It is the feminine of the Old Norse Brandr that means 'sword that was brought to Britain' during the Middle Ages.

**Freja**: This girl name is of Swedish, Old Norse, and Danish origins. It means 'like a lady'. It is very popular in Scandinavia but rare elsewhere. It is derived from the element *Freyja* meaning 'lady'. This name belongs to the goddess of death, war, beauty, and love in Norse mythology. She said most of the heroes that were slain were brought to her realm in Folkvangr. With her father Njord and brother Freyr. Some connect her to the goddess Frigg. In Denmark and Sweden, it is spelled Freja. In Norway, it is spelled Froja.

**Ingrid**: This girl name is of Old Norse origin and means 'beautiful goddess'. Ing was another name for

Freyr in Norse mythology. She was an important god of fertility, weather, and farming. Ingrid is an extremely popular name in the Scandinavian countries

**Ragna**: This girl name is of Swedish, Old Norse, and Danish origins and means 'giving advice'. This is a shortened form of Old Norse names that began with element 'regin' meaning 'counsel or advice'.

**Sigfrid**: This girl name is of Old Norse and Norwegian origins and means 'marvelous victory'. It is a variation of Sigrid. It is derived from the elements *sigr* meaning 'victory' and *fridr* meaning 'fair or beautiful'.

**Thora**: This girl name is of Old Norse origin and means 'like thunder'. It is the feminine form or Thor who is the Norse god of thunder, power, and war. Thora was a wife of Ragnar Lodbrok who was a king of Denmark in Norse mythology.

**Tyra**: This girl name is of Old Norse origin and means 'like thunder'. It is the feminine form of Tyr who is the Norse god of justice and war.

## Unisex

**Beau**: This unisex name is of French origin and means 'beautiful person'. It was used as a form of endearment for a girl or a nickname for a good man.

**Dagny**: This unisex name is of Old Norse origin and means 'new day started'. It is derived from the elements *dagr* meaning 'day' and *ny* meaning 'new'.

**Haley**: This unisex name is of English origin and means 'meadow of hay'. It is a variant of Haley. It is derived from Old English surname. It comes from *heg* meaning 'hay' and *leah* meaning 'clearing'. It could mean 'heroine' in the Old Norse language.

**Karina**: This unisex name is of Swedish, Russian, Polish, Norwegian, Greek, and Danish origins. It means pure or chaste. It is one of the most popular names with many different spellings over the entire world. It could be a variation of Katherine.

**Loki**: This unisex name is of Old Norse origin and means 'trickster'. Loki is the name of the trickster god in Norse mythology. He used fire and magic against people. He became very evil, and the other gods chained him to a rock. It is used as a nickname for someone who is thought to be a cheater.

**Mikko**: This unisex name is of Hebrew and Finnish origins and means 'which man is like God'? It is a variant of Michael. Can be spelled, Mika.

**Montana**: This unisex name is of Latin origin and means from 'a hilly land'. It is derived from a Spanish word that means 'mountain'. It is also used as a surname.

**Rayne**: This unisex name is of English origin and means 'woman of rain'. Could be based on the French word *reine* that means 'queen'.

**Signy**: This unisex name is of Danish, Norwegian, and Swedish origins and means 'latest victory'. It is derived from elements *sigr* meaning 'victory' and *ny* meaning 'new'. In Norse legends, it was the wife of Siggeir and the sister of Sigmund.

**Ziv**: This unisex name is of Hebrew origin and means 'shining'. It is the ancient name of a month in the Jewish calendar.

# German

## Boys

**Anton**: This boy name is of German origin. It is from the Roman name *Antonius*. The most memorable person within the Roman family was Marcus Antonius who ruled the Roman Empire with Augustus. When their friendship went south, his mistress Cleopatra and he were attacked, and they forced them to commit suicide, as stated in Shakespeare's tragedy, *Antony and Cleopatra*.

**Barney**: This boy name is of German origin. It is a shortened version of Bernard. It is derived from the element *bern* meaning 'bear' and *hard* meaning 'hardy or brave'. The Normans were the one who brought it to England, and it replaced the Old English name Beornheard. Several saints bore the name Bernard. Saint Bernard of Menthon built hospices in the 900s in the Swiss Alps. Saint Bernard of Clairvaux was a doctor of the church and a theologian in the 1300s.

**Conrad**: This boy name is of German origin. It is derived from the elements *kuoni* meaning 'brave' and *rad* meaning 'counsel'. A bishop and saint who lived in the 900s in Konstanz that is located in southern Germany. Several medieval Kings and Dukes bore this name as well. It was used some time during the Middle Ages in England but has become more common in the 1800s when Germany reintroduced the name.

**Dirk**: This boy name is of German origin. It is from the German name Theodoric meaning 'ruler of the people'. It is derived from the elements *theud* meaning 'people' and *ric* meaning 'ruler or power'. Theodoric the Great who was a king in the 500s of Ostrogoth and became ruler of Italy. His name became Romanized and was recorded as Theodoricus. The Gothic spelling is Diudreiks.

**Ferdinand**: This boy name is of German origin. It comes from Ferdinando which is the Old Spanish form of the Germanic name with the elements *fardi* meaning 'journey' and *nand* meaning 'brave or daring'. The Visigoths brought it to the Iberian Peninsula where royal families of Portugal and Spain began using it. It was popular with the Roman Empire, the Habsburg royal family, and Austria.

**Hans**: This boy name is of Scandinavian, Dutch, and German origins. It is a shortened version of Johannes. Johannes is from the Latin Ioannes meaning John. John is from the Hebrew name Yochanan meaning 'Yahweh is gracious'.

**Jansen**: This boy name is of Flemish, Low German, and Dutch origins. It was a surname meaning 'son of Jan'. It is derived from the name Johannes.

**Kiefer**: This boy name is of German origin. It is an occupational name for an overseer of wine cellars from the elements *kuofe* meaning 'barrel or vat'. It is also a version of the Middle High German *kiffen* 'to quarrel' and became a nickname for a person who likes to bicker. It is from the German *kiefer* meaning 'pine tree'. It is derived from two elements *kein* and *forhe* both meaning 'pine tree'.

**Leo**: This boy name is of German origin. It is derived from the Latin *leo* meaning 'lion' which is a version of Leon. It became popular with Christians as it was the name of 13 popes.

**Pepin**: This boy name is of German origin. It was originally a surname in northwest Germany around the city of Cologne. It is derived from the word *pepin* or *pipin* meaning 'seed of a fruit' and is an occupational name for a 'grower of fruit trees or gardener'.

## Girls

**Adalie**: This girl name is of German origin. It means 'noble one' or 'God is my refuge'. It is a variation of Adalia which is Old German and Hebrew. It is also a variation of Adela which is Old German.

**Bernadette**: This girl name is of German origin. It is a feminine version of the name Bernard. It comes from the Germanic element *bern* meaning 'bear' combined with *hard* meaning 'hardy or brave'. The Normans introduced it to England, and it replaced *Beornheard*.

**Delmira**: This girl name is of German origin. It means 'famous or noble'. It is a variation of Delma and has the nickname of Adelma.

**Farica**: This girl name is of German origin and means 'peaceful ruler'. It is a shortened version of Frederica. It is made up of the elements *frid* meaning 'peace' and *ric* meaning 'power or ruler'. This name is common in German speaking regions.

**Geneva**: This girl name is of German origin. It comes from the medieval name *Genovefa*. It is derived from the elements *kuni* meaning 'family' or 'kin' and *wefa* meaning 'woman or wife'. Another origin is Gaulish from the Celtic element *genos* meaning 'family or kin'.

**Georgia**: This girls name is a variation of the German name, Georgina, which is the feminine version of the name, George. The word was derived from the Greek word *georgos*, which means 'farmer or earthworker'. The name became popular in England when the German-born George I took the British throne.

**Jenell**: The name Jenell is a German name which means 'kindness, knowledge, and understanding'. In Latin and English, the name means 'maiden' and is a variation of the name, Janelle.

**Joli**: This name comes from French origins. While in France it is not often given as a given name. The name means 'beautiful' in French and 'pretty and cheerful' in English.

**Katrina**: The name Katrina is a variation of Katherine. It is derived from the Greek name *Aikaterine*. It is debated as to where this name originally came from. It could be the Greek name *Hekaterine*, which was taken from *hekateros*, which means 'each of the two'. And it's also believed to have come from the Goddess Hecate.

**Lorelei**: This name comes from a Germanic name that means 'luring rock'. The name is derived from a rocky headland that is located on the Rhine River.

# Unisex

**Ade**: The name Ade is a variation of the German name, Adalwold, which means 'noble wolf'. Broken down, it comes from the element *adal* meaning 'noble' and wulf meaning 'wolf'. It was a popular name among Swedish Kings.

**Al**: This name mainly started out as a nickname for somebody named Albert, but has since become a popular choice for a given name. It comes from the German name Adalbert, which is made up of the element *adal*, meaning 'noble' and 'beraht' meaning *bright*. This was a common medieval German royalty name.

**Bernie**: The name Bernie comes from the name Bernard. The name was derived from the Germanic element *bern* meaning 'bear' and mixed with *hard* meaning 'brave and hardy'.

**Claiborne**: Not much is known about this name. It has origins in both Germany and England. In German, it means 'boundary with clover'. It's a common English surname that was found in the Norfolk and southeast area of England, possibly meaning 'clay by a river'.

**Clovis**: This name is a shortened version of the name *Clodovicus*, which is the Latinized form of the German name *Chlodevech*, which is also changed to Ludwig. It comes from the elements *hlud* meaning 'famous' and *wig* which means 'battle or war'.

**Fritzi**: This name comes from a diminutive form of the German name, Friederike, which comes from the name, Frederick. The name means 'peaceful ruler'. It comes from the elements *frid* meaning 'peace' and *ric* meaning 'power or ruler'.

**Halle**: The name Halle came about from the German surname, Halle, which is a 'cognate of Hall'. This name was derived from an Old English word, heal, which means 'hall or manor'. This name was given to a person that worked or lived in a manor.

**Karlyn**: This name has both English and Old German origins. Karlyn means 'free man' and is a variation of the Old German name, Carlene and the English name, Karleen.

**Malin**: This name a shorter variation of the name Magdalene. The name originated from a title that meant 'of Magdala'. The New Testament character Mary Magdalene was named such because she was from Magdala, which is a village on the Sea of Galilee.

**Rory**: The name Rory has become gained popularity as a German name over the past few centuries. The names origin is Gaelic. It comes from the Irish name, Ruairi, and the Scottish name, Ruairidah. The name means 'red king'.

# Historical

## Boys

**Amadeus**: The name Amadeus means 'love of God'. The name was derived from the Latin word *amare* which means 'to love' and *Deus* which means 'God'. The famous composer, Wolfgang Amadeus Mozart, carried this name.

**Aurelius**: This name is a common name from early saints. It started as a Roman family name and was derived from the Latin word *aureus* which means 'gilded or golden'.

**Cassius**: This name started out as a Roman family name that was probably derived from the Latin word *cassus* which means 'vain or empty'. This was also a common name given to saints.

**Demetrius**: This name is a Latin version of the Greek name, Demetrios, which came from the name of the Greek Goddess, Demeter. Many early saints were given this name, and Seleucid kingdom and the Kings of Macedon used this name.

**Felix**: This name is derived from a famous Roman cognomen, which means 'successful or lucky' in Latin. It was given as an agnomen to the 1st-century Roman general Sulla. In the New Testament, it belongs to the governor of Judea. This was a popular name for early Christians because of its meaning.

**Magnus**: This name is derived from a late Latin word that means 'great'. A 7th-century saint bore this name. It gained popularity in Scandinavia with the 11th century Norwegian King Magnus I.

**Septimus**: This name is a Roman given name, which in Latin it means 'seventh'. This name was given to the Emperor Septimus Severus, which was a patron of arts and letters.

**Severus**: This name is derived from a Roman family name, and in Latin it means 'stern'. This was a popular name among early saints.

**Thor**: This name comes from an Old Norse word which means 'thunder', which came from an early Germanic word. Thor is the god of thunder, storms, strength, and war in Norse mythology, and is the son of Odin.

**Urban**: The name Urban comes from the Latin name *Urbanus* which means 'city dweller'. Paul mentions this name in one of his New Testament epistles. It has been a name of eight popes.

## Girls

**Aeliana**: The name Aeliana is the female form of the name, Aelianus. Aelianus is a Roman cognomen which they derived from the name, Aelius. This family name was possibly taken from the Greek word *helios* which means 'the sun'.

**Atarah**: This name in Hebrew means crown. Atarah was the wife of Jerahmeel in the Old Testament.

**Crispina**: This name is the feminine form of the name Crispin. This was a Roman cognomen, Crispinus, which they got from the name, Crispus. A 3rd century Roman, Saint Crispin, was martyred along with his twin broth in Gaul. They are considered to be the patron saints of shoemakers.

**Delicia**: This name was either derived from the Latin word *deliciae* which means 'pleasure or delight' or the English word delicious. This name is a rarely used name and has only been popular since the early 20th century.

**Felicia**: The name Felicia is the female version of the Latin name, Felicius, which is derived from the name, Felix. It has occasionally been used in England since the Middle Ages.

**Jonet**: The name Jonet is an obsolete Scottish spelling of the name, Janet. Janet is a medieval version of the name, Jane, which is a feminine version of the name, John. The meaning of the name goes back to the Hebrew name, Yochanan, which means 'Yahweh is gracious'.

**Lucilla**: This name is the Latin diminutive of Lucia. A 3rd-century saint that was martyred in Rome had this name. The name is derived from the Latin word *lux* which means 'light'.

**Minerva**: This name is possibly derived from the Latin word *mens* which means 'intellect', but is more likely to have an Etruscan origin. In Roman mythology, Minerva was the goddess of war and wisdom, which is basically the equivalent of the Greek Goddess, Athena. It has been a popular name since after the English Renaissance.

**Sabina**: This name is the female version of Sabinus, which is a Roman cognomen that means 'Sabine' in Latin. Ancient people that lived in central Italy were known as the Sabines and their lands were taken by the Romans after many wars.

**Viviana**: The name, Viviana, is the female version of Vivianus. The 4th-century saint, Saint Viviana, was a martyr. The name was derived from the Latin word *vivus* which means 'alive'.

# Unisex

**Alva**: This unisex name is derived from the name, Alf. It comes from the Old Norse word *alfr* meaning 'elf'. The name could also be a variation of the name, Alvah, which in Hebrew means 'his highness'.

**Angel**: This name is derived from the Latin medieval masculine name, Angelus, which came from the name that was given to heavenly creature. That name came from the Greek word *angelos* which means 'messenger'. In the English-speaking world, it's not that popular.

**Brook**: The name, Brook, started as an English surname. The surname was given to people that lived near a brook, making the meaning of the name 'the one who lives near a brook' or 'a running stream'.

**Cheyenne**: This name comes from the Dakota word, shahiyena, which means 'red speakers'. This name comes from Native Americans who are from the Great Plains. The Dakotas gave the Cheyenne this name because their language was unrelated to theirs.

**Dee**: The name, Dee, in Welsh is often a nickname for a person considered swarthy, and comes from the Welsh word *du* meaning 'black or dark'. In Irish, it is a variation of Daw. In Scotland and England, it is a habitational name of a person that lived near the banks on the Dee River in Cheshire or in Scotland. Both of these were derived from a Celtic word that means goddess or sacred.

**Dusty**: This name was often given to people as a nickname if they seemed to be dusty. It is also a variation of Dustin. This name is derived from an English surname which came from the Old Norse name, Torsten, which means Thor's stone.

**Gale**: This name is a shortened version of the name Abigail, which comes from the Hebrew name 'Avigayil, which means 'my father is joy'. It also comes from an English surname that was taken from a Middle English word, gaile, which means 'jovial'.

**Jackie**: This name most often comes from the names Jacqueline or Jack. Jack is the medieval diminutive of John, which comes from the Hebrew name, Yochana, which means 'Yahweh is gracious'. Jacqueline is the feminine version of Jacques, which is the French form of the name, Jacob. The name means 'may God protect.

**Johnnie**: This name is a diminutive of the name, John. The name, John, comes the Latin word Johannes, which comes from the Greek name, Joannes, which comes from the Hebrew name *Yochanan*, which means 'Yahweh is gracious'.

**Lee**: The name Lee started out as a surname that was derived from an Old English word leah, which means 'clearing'. Lee means 'dweller by the wood or clearing'. Lee is commonly used in combination names like Lee-Ann and Bobby-Lee.

# Most Common

## Boys

**Alexander**: This name is the Latinized form of the Greek name, Alexandros. This name means 'defending men', which comes from the Greek word *alexo* meaning 'to defend, help' and *aner* meaning 'man'. This was also another name for the hero Paris in Greek mythology.

**Benjamin**: The name Benjamin comes from the Hebrew name *Binyamin*. It means 'son of the right hand' or 'son of the south'. In the Old Testament, the youngest son of Jacob was Benjamin and a founder of a southern Hebrew tribe.

**Carter**: The name Carter started out being used for the surname of a cart driver. It is of English descent and it means 'Driver of a cart'.

**Cole**: The origin of this name is Anglo-Saxon. This name came from a surname that in Old English was the byname Cola. This name means charcoal and used to be given to people that had dark features.

**Daniel**: The name Daniel originates from the old Hebrew name *Daniyyel,* which means 'God is my judge'. In the Old Testament, Daniel is a Hebrew prophet. The name became popular during the Middle Ages in England due to the biblical character.

**Dylan**: This name comes from Wales, and it's derived from the element *dy,* which means 'great' and *llanw* which means 'tide and flow'. Dylan, in Welsh mythology, was a hero or god that was associated with the sea.

**Greyson**: This name is a variation of the English name Grayson. It comes from an English surname that meant 'son of the steward'. This name was derived from the Middle English word, *greyve*, which means 'steward'.

**Jackson**: The name Jackson started out as an English surname that means 'son of Jack'. In English, Jack is the diminutive form of John.

**Jacob**: This name originated from the Latin word *Iacobus* which was derived from the Greek word *Iakobos*, which was derived from the Hebrew name *Ya'aqov*. Jacob in the Old Testament is the son of Rebecca and Isaac. During the Middle Ages in England, Jacob was viewed as a mainly Jewish name. It started being used as a Christian name after the Protestant Reformation.

**Juan**: This name is the Manx and Spanish version of the name Johannes, which is the name, John. The name John dates back to the Hebrew name *Yochanan*, which means 'Yahweh is gracious'.

**Matthew**: This name is an English form of the word Matthaios, which is a Greek form of a Hebrew name, *Mattityahu,* which means 'gift of Yahweh'. In the Bible Matthew is one of the 12 apostles.

**Miles**: This name comes from the Germanic name, Milo. The name was introduced to England by the

Normans in the form of the name, Miles. The actual definition of the name is not certain. It may be connected with the Slavic element *milu* which means 'gracious'. It could also date back to the Latin word miles, meaning soldier.

**Oliver**: This name is derived from the Norman French name Olivier, which was a form of a Germanic name Alfher, or the Norse name, Olaf. The spelling of the name was changed over time because of its association with the Latin word *olive* which means 'olive tree'.

**Roman**: The name Roman comes from a late Latin name *Romanus*, which means 'Roman'. The name Roman means to be of Rome.

**Samuel**: Samuel comes from the Hebrew name S*hemu'el* which may mean "God has heard' or 'name of God'. Samuel, in the Old Testament, was the last ruling judge. Samuel becomes a popular Christian name after the Protestant Reformation.

**Theodore**: This name originated from the Greek name Theodoros, which means 'gift of God.' It is broken down into the Greek words *theos* meaning God and *doron* meaning gift.

**Tristan**: This name comes from the French form of the Pictish name, Drustan, which is also a diminutive form of Drust. The name's spelling has been changed because of the Latin *tristis* which means sad.

**Vincent**: The name Vincent comes from the Roman name, Vincentius, which comes from the Latin *vincere* which means 'to conquer'. This was a very popular name for the early Christians, and many saints bore this name.

**Wesley**: This English name comes from an old surname that was derived from a place name that, in Old English, means 'west meadow'. At one time, the name was given in honor of the Methodist faith founder, John Wesley.

**Weston**: This name is of English origin. It started out as a surname that was given to people who lived west of the town. It comes from an Old English word.

## Girls

**Aurora**: The name Aurora comes from a Latin word that means dawn. In Roman mythology, Aurora was the Goddess of the morning. It has been used as a name since the Renaissance

**Chloe**: The name Chloe means 'green shoot' in Greek, which refers to the new plants that grow in spring. The Greek Goddess Demeter used this as an epithet. The name is also mentioned in the New Testament in one of Paul's epistles.

**Daisy**: This is an English name that was taken from the pretty white flower. It was originally derived from the Old English word *dægeseage* which means 'day eye'. The word first appeared as a given name during the 1800s, which was also at the same time as many other flowers and plants were given names.

**Elizabeth**: This name was derived from the Greek name, Elisabet, which was derived from the Hebrew name *Elisheva* which means 'my God is abundance' or 'my God is an oath'. In the Old Testament, the Hebrew version of the name appears where Elisheba is the wife of Aaron. The Greek form makes an appearance in the New Testament where John the Baptist's mother is Elizabeth.

**Evelyn**: The name Evelyn comes from an English surname, which came from Aveline; a given name. When the name was first used as a given name in the 17th century, it was used more often for boys.

**Grace**: This name comes from the English word grace, which was originated from the Latin word *gratia*. The Puritans created this name in the 17th century as one of their virtue names.

**Harmony**: This is an English name that was derived from the English word harmony. The word was originally derived from the Greek word *harmonia*. Within Greek mythology, Harmonia is the Goddess of harmony, happy marriages, sisterhood, and brotherhood. Her parents are Ares, god of war, and Aphrodite, goddess of love. Harmony is a musical term that signifies a note combination that is played at the same time that gives a pretty melody.

**Hannah**: This name originates with the Hebrew name, Channah, which means 'grace or favor'. In the Old Testament, Elkanah's wife had this name. Hannah didn't become a common name until after the Protestant Reformation.

**Katherine**: This name comes from the Greek name Aikaterine. It is debated as to where it originated and is believed could have come from an early Greek name *hekaterine*, which means each of the two, or from the Goddess, Hecate. It may also be from the Greek word *aikia*, which means torture, or it may also be from the Coptic name that means 'my consecration of your name.' Early Christians associated the name with the Greek word *katharos*, which means pure.

**Kimberly**: The name Kimberly comes from a city in South Africa, named, Kimberley. This city was named after Lord Kimberley. The name is a variation of Cyneburg, which means royal fortress. Broken down, it comes from the Old English cyne, which means royal, and burg, meaning fortress.

**Layla**: This name comes from an Arabic word meaning night. The 7th-century poems, Layla was the romantic interest of a poet known as Qays. This became a popular romance within medieval Persia and Arabia.

**Lily**: This name is derived from the Latin word *lilium*. The name comes from the flower, which is a symbol of purity.

**Madison**: This name started out as an English surname, which means 'son of Maud'. The name became a popular name for girls when the 1984 movie "Splash" came out.

**Maria**: This name is the Latin form of the Greek name *Mapiaz*, which comes from the Hebrew name

Mary. Maria is the most common form of the name Mary in most European languages and the secondary form in many other languages like English. In some countries, Maria is used as a masculine middle name. The meaning is not completely known, but it could mean 'wished for child,' 'sea of bitterness,' or 'rebelliousness.' But it is most likely taken from an Egyptian name, broken down to *mry*, meaning beloved, or *mr*, meaning love.

**Melanie**: This name comes from Mélanie, which is the French version of the Latin Melania, which they derived from the Greek word melaina, which means dark or black. A 5th-century Roman saint was given this name; she gave all of her money to charity. It became a popular name during the Middle Ages in France.

**Rachel**: The name Rachel is derived from the Hebrew name Rachel, which means ewe. This is the favorite wife of Jacob in the Old Testament, and she is the mother of Benjamin, and Joseph. She was also Jacob's first wife, Leah's, little sister. This was a common name for Jews during the Middle Ages, but it didn't become a Christian name until after the Protestant Reformation.

**Rose**: This name started out as a Norman form of a German name, which was made up of *hruod*, which means 'fame', and *heid*, which means 'type, kind, and sort'. The English was introduced to this name by the Normans in the forms of Rohese and Roese. From early on it has been associated with the good smelling flower rose, which came from the Latin word *rosa*. When the name became popular again in the 19th century, it was probably due to the flower.

**Scarlett**: This name came from the surname that they used for a person that made or sold clothes that had been made from scarlet, which is a type of cloth. This name was derived from the Persian word *saghrilat*.

**Valerie**: This name is the German and English version of Valeria and Czech version of Valérie. The name Valeria is the female form of Valerius, which comes from the Latin word *valere*, which means 'to be strong'. Many early saints bore this name.

**Victoria**: In Latin, this name means victory, and is borne of the Roman Goddess of victory. This name is the female version of the name, Victorius. The first use of this name was from a North African martyr and saint of the 4th century.

## Unisex

**Alex**: This name is a shortened version of any name that begins with Alex. Lately, it has become popular as a given name for both boys and girls, instead of just used as a nickname. The name means 'to defend or help'.

**Drew**: The name Drew is derived from the name Andrew, which is the English version of the Greek Andreas, which they derived from *andreios*, which means 'manly and masculine'. Andre was the first disciple of Jesus in the New Testament.

**Jaden**: The name Jaden is a recently invented name, became popular in the 1990s, and used the popular aden suffix that is found in many other names. It is also, sometimes, considered to be derived from the name Jadon which means 'he will judge' or 'thankful' in Hebrew.

**Jordan**: This name comes from the name of the river that runs between Israel and Jordan. The name comes from the Hebrew word, Yarden, and it was derived from *yarad* which means 'flow down or descend'. Jesus Christ was baptized in the river by John the Baptist.

**Kyle**: While this name is seen more for boys, it has recently become popular for both sexes. It originated from the Scottish surname that was derived from the Gaelic word *caol,* which means 'strait, channel, or narrow'.

**Parker**: This name originated in England as an occupational surname for people. It means 'keeper of the park'.

**Nico**: The name Nico comes from the name Nicholas or Nicodemus. It's derived from the Greek name *Nikolaos* which means 'victory of the people'. This is broken down into the Greek word *nike* which means 'victory' and *laos* which means 'people'.

**Regan**: This name is believed to have Celtic origins, but the meaning is unknown. Shakespeare used the name in his play "King Lear" which is found in early British legends. Regan also comes from the name

Reagan, which is an Irish surname and an Anglicized form of *Ó Riagain* which means 'descendant of Riagan'.

**Sawyer**: This name comes from a Middle English surname that was an occupational name meaning 'sawer of wood'. This name is probably most popular in the book *The Adventures of Tom Sawyer* by Mark Twain.

**Skyler**: The name Skyler is derived from the name *Schuyler*. The change in the spelling happened because of the name Tyler and the word sky. In Dutch, *Schuyler* is a surname that means 'scholar'.

# Most Unusual

## Boys

**Ace**: This unique name is typically given to people as a nickname. It originated from an English word that means 'highest rank'. The English word was derived from a Latin word that means 'first-rate or unity'.

**Axel**: The name Axel is a Medieval Danish form of the name, Absalon. Absalom comes from the Hebrew name, Avshalom, which means 'my father is peace'. Within the Old Testament, Absolom is the son of King David.

**Constantine**: This name comes from the Latin name *Constantinus*, and is derived from *Constans*. The Roman Emperor Constantine the Great was the first emperor to adopt Christianity. He took the empire to Byzantium and renamed it Constantinople, which has been renamed to Istanbul.

**Finn**: Finn comes from Irish origin and is an older form of *Fionn*. The name means 'white or fair'. Finn is the most common Anglicized form.

**Gunner**: This name is derived from the Scandinavian name, Gunther, which means 'bold warrior'. This comes from the Old Norse name *Gunnar* which was derived from the word *gunnr* which means 'battle, strife, and war'.

**Jett**: The name Jett comes from the English word, Jet. This name can refer to the flying aircraft of the same name or a black mineral or color.

**Kane**: The name Kane is derived from the Irish name, Cathan. Cathan came from the Gaelic word *cath* which means 'battle'. In Hawaii and Japan, the name is transformed into a two-syllable name pronounced, KA-ned. In Welsh, it means 'beautiful', in Japanese, it means 'golden', and in Hawaiian, it means 'man of the Eastern sky.'

**Rocco**: This name is Germanic, and was derived from the element *hrok* which means 'rest'. This is the same name of a 14th-century French saint that helped nurse plague victims but ended up contracting it as well. He is now considered the patron saint of the sick.

**Titus**: This name is a Roman given name that comes from unknown meaning, but it could be related to the Latin word *titulus* which means 'title of honor'. A more likely origin is Oscan, since the name come from the legendary Sabine King, Titus Tatius.

**Zane**: The origin of this name is Semitic, where it is a variation of Jon which means 'God's gracious gift.' Another meaning of the word is 'good' when used in this masculine form.

## Girls

**Addilyn**: This girl name is French in origin and comes from the names, Adeline and Adele, which mean 'kind and noble'. Addilyn can also be a variation of the name Madelyn, which in France came from Madeleine which was in honor of Mary Magdalene.

**Aria**: The origin of this pretty girl name is Italian where it means 'literally, air, or melody and song'. Aria is a vocal solo which is typically performed during operas. It has only been used as a name since the 20th century.

**Bronwyn**: This name has both Irish and Welsh origins. The Welsh feminine version is spelled Bronwen, while the Irish feminine version is spelled Bronwyn. Both versions mean 'pure and dark', 'white breasted', and 'white breast'.

**Camari**: This name comes from Gaelic origins. Originally a surname that meant 'crooked nose', broken down it comes from *cam* which means 'crooked' and *sron* which means 'nose'. This is the same as the name Cameron.

**Diem**: The origin of Diem is Latin, and means 'day'. In Vietnamese, the name means 'pretty'.

**Effie**: Effie is of Scottish origin. It comes from the Anglicized form of the word *Oighrig*, which means 'new speckled one'.

**Ember**: The name Ember comes for the Old English word *œmyrge*, which comes from the proto-Germanic word *aima* meaning 'ashes'. The word Ember means 'glowing coal in a dying fire.' This given name was first recorded in the 1800s, which most likely came as a transfer of the surname, Ember.

**Fleur**: The origin of Fleur comes from a French word meaning 'flower'. Fleur was introduced to the English through the author, John Galsworthy, who gave it to a character in his books.

**Gianna**: This unique girl's name is a feminized version of the Latin name, John. The origin of Gianna comes from Italy as a diminutive of Giovanna. It means 'the Lord is gracious'.

**Harlyn**: Harlyn is the feminized version of the name, Harlan. The name originated from an Old English surname that means 'hare land'.

**Imogen**: Imogen likely originated from the Gaelic word, inghean, which means maiden. Shakespeare gave the princess in *Cymbeline* this name, and he based her on the character, Innogen.

**Lilith**: The name Lilith is derived from the Akkadian word, lilitu, which means 'of the night'. This is the same name as the demon in the ancient Assyrian myths. In the Jewish faith, she was Adam's first wife who was expelled from Eden and then replaced by Eve because Lilith was not willing to submit to him. The offspring that Lilith and Adam produced were the evil spirits.

**Mavis**: The name Mavis comes from Old French origin, and is the name of a bird. The bird is also referred to as a song thrush. The first 'person' that was ever given this name was one of the characters in Marie Corelli's book *The Sorrows of Satan*.

**Naya**: The origin of Naya comes from Arabic where it means 'new'. It is also a form of the names, Naia and Nia.

**Ophelia**: This name is derived from the Greek word *ophelos* which means 'help'. Jacopo Sannazaro, a 15th-century poet, is probably the one who created this name in his poem "Arcadia". Shakespeare then borrowed the name in his play "Hamlet".

**Trinity**: Trinity is an English name that is given in honor of Christian beliefs that God is one essence, but has three expressions: Father, Son, and Holy Spirit. Trinity only became a given name in the 20th century.

**Uri**: The name Uri is of Biblical and Hebrew origins. In the Old Testament, this was the name of the father, Bezalel. The meaning of the name is 'my fire or my light'.

## Unisex

**Ainsley**: This unisex name is from Gaelic origin and began life as a Scottish surname, which was taken from the home name of Ainsley. This name was derived from element name *Ægen's* or *Æne's*, as well as the Old English *Leah*, which means 'enclosure, meadow, clearing, or wood'.

**Arlo**: There are many different origins for this unisex name. In Old English, it's believed to have come from the Anglo-Saxon word *here* meaning 'war, troops, fortified, and army' and the word *hlaw* meaning 'fortified hill, cairn, and mound'. From Italian origin, it is derived from the names, Karlos, Carlos, which is a variant of the English name, Charles.

**August**: Month names have come in and out of popularity, and August has recently hit a stride as a popular unisex name. August originates from the German form of the Latin word Augustus. It means 'to be venerable, majestic, or dignity'.

**Blaine**: The unisex name Blaine is believed to have Gaelic origins. In most translations, Blaine means either 'lean or thin', in certain translations it means 'yellow' or 'the source of a river'.

**Bodhi**: This unisex name comes from 'the tree that Buddha sat under,' which is where he gained his enlightenment. Bodhi is a Sanskrit word which means enlightenment or awakening. The Bodhi tree is a big fig tree. As opposed to some other spiritual and religious names, Bodhi has a more friendly and upbeat meaning.

**Braidy**: This name is a fun twist on Brady with Irish and Old English origin. The definition is a bit unclear, ranging from broad-chested to broad-eyed to a broad island. Broad is the one word that ties them all together. In Old English it came from the elements *brad* meaning 'broad' and *eage* meaning 'eye'.

**Carson**: This unisex name comes from Scottish and Middle English origin. It is a transferred use of a surname which means 'Carr's son'. In Scottish origin, it means 'carre', which is mossy place or marsh, and car. In Welsh, it means 'caer' which is a fort, and in Gaelic, it means 'carr' which is a rock.

**Cody**: Cody comes from the Gaelic surname *Ó Cuidighthigh*, which means to be a 'descendant of Cuidightheach'. Cody also has the meaning of 'helpful or pillow'.

**Cohen**: This unisex name is a very common Jewish surname that is believed to mean priest. As a surname, Cohen is royal name in the Jewish faith. Some may be unaware of the meaning behind the name and find it cool sounding for a first name. Some religious groups may find it offensive if used as a first name.

**Dallas**: While it may be a Texas City, it has origins in Scotland, meaning 'a meadow dwelling'. It is derived from the Gaelic word *dail* which means 'field' and *eas* which means 'waterfall'.

**Dana**: Dana comes from many different origins. One such meaning is to come from 'Dame' meaning Denmark. Dana is also another form of the name *Danu* which is a Celtic goddess of fertility. In Persia, the name means 'knowledgeable'.

**Darian**: The meaning of Darian is 'upholder of the good'. The name has Persian routes. Darian is a variation of Darius which is a royal Persian name.

**Devon**: Devon is a derivation of the Irish name Devin, which is derived from the Gaelic word *damh* which means 'a poet'. Devon means 'a defender'. It is also believed to be derived from the name of an English county, Devon. This county received its name from the Celtic tribe, Dumnonii.

**Dian**: Dian comes from many origins. In French, Dian means 'the divine'. In German, it comes from mythology that means 'from the God of wine.' In Indonesian, it means a 'candle'. Depending on the country and culture, Dian has several different meanings.

**Emery**: This unisex name was introduced to the English by the Normans and is still a rare name to hear. Emery is the Norman form of Emmerich. The name survived through the Middle Ages, and most of the modern use of it has been inspired by the surname, Emery. The name has different meanings such as 'power, universal, work, and home'.

**Hadley**: Hadley originated from an English surname which means 'heather field'. Hadley has always been a unisex name. Another meaning for Hadley is 'Heath near the wasteland'.

**Harlow**: Harlow originated from an Old English surname that had been derived from a place name known as *hœr* meaning 'rock' or the word *here* meaning 'army' which was combined with the word *hlaw* meaning 'hill'.

**Haven**: This unisex name originates from an English word that means 'safe place'. It ultimately came from the Old English word 'hœfen'. This is a great name for parents that don't want to go as far as heaven.

**Indiana**: This unisex name comes from the American state, Indiana, which means 'land of the Indians'. In England, it also means the country of India.

**Indigo**: This name comes from the English word indigo, which refers to the purplish-blue dye or color. The word originally was derived from the Greek word

*Indikon* which means 'Indic, from India'.

**Jaya**: The name Jaya is derived from a Sanskrit word that means 'victory'. This came from a transcription of the feminine form of the Hindu Goddess, Durga and the masculine form of several Hindu text characters. As a modern name, in Southern India, it is used as both male and female but in the North it is more commonly female.

**Jazz**: Jazz is a great unisex name if you are a fan of the music, but as a name, it originated from the name Jasmine. Jasmine is a tropical plant that is commonly used in teas and perfumes.

**Jersey**: The meaning of this unisex name is Grassy Island. The name originated from the English culture where it originated. Jersey is a Channel Island off of the UK coast, as well as Guernsey.

**Kai**: The unisex name, Kai, is a Hawaiian word meaning sea. Kai in Mandarin Chinese has several meanings such as 'victory' and 'open'. In Japanese, Kai has the meaning of 'ocean, recovery, shell, and restoration'.

**Lane**: Lane comes from an English surname that means 'from the narrow road'. The surname originated with a person that lived close to a lane.

**Marlow**: This name comes from an Old English word which means driftwood. The very first phrase literally meant 'lake leavings'. It soon became a place name in Buckinghamshire, England, and then changed to a surname that was given to families that lived in that area.

**Misha**: There are two different meanings and origins for the name, Misha. One is Hebrew which means 'who resembles God?' The other is Russian which is the pet form of Michael.

**Neo**: In Africa, this unisex name means gift and in English, the name means 'new'. Neo is of Greek origin.

**Orion**: This unisex name comes from Greek origin meaning 'the hunter or son of fire'. In Roman and Greek mythology, Orion was Poseidon's son. He was loved by Diana, a goddess, but accidentally died at her hands. He was then placed in the heavens as the constellation.

**Penn**: This unisex name is of English origin, and is a more popular surname than given name. The meaning of Penn is 'enclosure or corral'.

**Phoenix**: This name comes from Greek and Egyptian mythology referring to a beautiful and immortal bird. After the bird lived many centuries in the Arabian Desert, the bird would be overtaken by fire and then rise out of its own ashes. This cycle would repeat every 500 years. The name derived from the Greek word *Phoinix* which means 'dark red'.

**Quinn**: Quinn comes from an Irish surname, which is an Anglicized version of *Ó Cuinn*, which means 'descendant of Conn'. The name was derived from the word *conn* which means 'intelligence, wisdom, or reason'.

**Remy**: The name Remy is a French form of Remigius, a Latin name. The Latin name was derived from the Latin word *remigis* meaning 'oarsman'.

**Rowan**: Rowan is a name that was derived from an Irish surname that is an Anglicized version of *Ó Ruadhain* which means 'descendant of Ruadhan'. Another origin of this name is from the rowan tree.

**Sage**: The name sage originated from Latin where sage refers to a plant that is seen by many to have special cleansing and healing properties. It can also refer to a person that is seen as very wise.

**Shae**: Shae is of Gaelic origin, and it means 'to be admirable'. It comes from the Anglicized form of the word *seaghdha*.

**Storm**: The name storm comes from the Old English word, storm, and it also originated from the Old Norse word *stormr*.

**Val**: Val comes from the name Valentine, which originated from the Roman cognomen Valentinus. This originated from the name Valens, which means 'healthy, strong, and vigorous'.

**Ziv**: Ziv is a Hebrew unisex name that means 'radiant and bright'. This is the same name as the second month of the Jewish calendar.

# Conclusion

Thanks for making it through to the end of *Baby Names: The Ultimate Book of Baby Names – Includes the Latest Trends, Meanings, Origins and Spiritual Significance*. Let's hope it was informative and able to provide you with all of the tools you need to achieve your goals of picking the best baby name.

The next thing is to make the hard decision of picking only one name for your little bundle of joy.

Finally, if you found this book useful in any way, a review on Amazon is always appreciated!

# Newborn 101

*The Essential Guide for New Parents to Raise a Healthy Baby*

# Table of Contents

# Introduction

Congratulations on downloading this book and thank you for doing so.

The following chapters will discuss some of the topics that new mothers want to know about when bringing home their newborns. This is an exciting time in your life, and you are ready to bring home that little baby and start your new life with them. But despite all of this excitement and your happiness, it can still be a time of concerns. Mothers may be worried about how to breastfeed, how to get through labor, how they can prepare for the baby, how to take care of their baby when they first bring the newborn home and so much more.

It is perfectly natural to ask all of these questions and being prepared ahead of time can make it easier to take care of your baby later on. This guidebook will provide you with some of the answers you need to properly take care of your newborn. We will talk about how to prepare your home, the stages of labor, how to make breastfeeding easier, ways to soothe your baby when they are fussy, and even when it is time to call the doctor over one of your concerns.

Every new parent has questions and concerns about taking care of their babies. With the help of this guidebook, you will have all of the information that you need to gain confidence so you can spend less time worrying and more time bonding with your new baby.

There are plenty of books on this subject on the market, thanks again for choosing this one! Every effort was made to ensure it is full of as much useful information as possible, please enjoy!

# Chapter 1: How to Prepare Your Home

You can even start preparing yourself and your home before the baby arrives. This is the perfect time to get a head start on some cleaning, baby proofing and organizing before you have those sleepless nights and a baby to take care of. Taking care of some of the essentials ahead of time can help you to remain calm once the baby comes home because you won't have so many worries running through your head. Here are a few of the things that you can do to help prepare yourself and your home for your new baby.

## Feed yourself

Once you bring home that baby, there isn't going to be a lot of time for preparing meals, and you don't necessarily want to spend a lot of money going out all of the time. Preparing ahead of time so you and your family will have food for the first few weeks is important to ensure that you stay healthy and have the energy that you need.

There are a few ways that you can do it. You can purchase some freezer meals to have on hand for when you are too tired to cook. You can prepare some of your own freezer meals as well, which is a lot healthier and will even save you money. Some families will purchase a few gift cards so they can grab something easy when they feel hungry.

## Feed the baby

If you are choosing to breastfeed your baby, make sure that you purchase a high-quality pump. You can either purchase one (many insurance companies will help with this now), or you can rent a hospital grade one. Consider a nursing pillow as well because this will make both you and the baby more comfortable. Even with breastfeeding, consider having some bottles on hand for when you send the baby to daycare, or you are interested in letting others feed the baby at times.

## Try to get some sleep

This one is easier said than done in most cases, but getting enough rest, especially when this is your first baby and you don't have others to chase around, is so important. Many mothers during the last trimester have trouble getting enough sleep because they are uncomfortable, they may have aches and pains, or the baby is moving around a lot. But even just taking it easy will help you out and prepare you for when the baby comes.

It will not be long before your baby arrives, and the long days and nights will start to catch up to you. It is best to get as much sleep as possible during this time, but taking things slowly, such as not working out as hard, taking some time off work, and just relaxing at night, can make things so much easier to handle and will rest your body up before baby gets here.

## Setting up the baby's room

Take some time to set up the room for your baby. Whether you are keeping the baby in their own room or in your room for a bit, there are a few things that you can do. Start out by making the room a little bit darker. The baby will take naps during the day, but this can be hard when the room is bright and sunny. You can get some light canceling curtains to help and keep some lights inside of the room down to a minimum. Having some white noise or soft music in the room can be nice as well.

In addition to making sure that the room is comfy and dark for a sleeping time, you also can organize some other things. Hang up and put away the clothes that you have gotten for the baby. Set up the crib and make sure that the sheets are on properly. Store the other supplies that you have gotten such as diapers, bath supplies, wipes, toys, book and more. Get everything organized ahead of time to help put you at ease.

## Smooth out the edges

Edges need to be taken care of before the baby is born. If there are any edges that you are worried about, it is time to smooth them out. This can be on the sides of walls, on door frames, on furniture and so on. Take a few moments to go through the house and see where some of the edges are. Imagine how you would feel if you ran into one of these, and then determine if you would like to smooth them out.

These edges are going to be dangerous once your little one starts moving around, which will be sooner than you can imagine, so take care of those edges before the baby arrives.

## Secure moveable furniture

Take a look around your home and see if any pieces of furniture can easily be moved. Do they shake a bit and would they be an issue if the baby started grabbing onto them when they begin walking? If there is any furniture that can move around or topple, it is time to secure it properly. Make sure that shelving is hooked up to the wall, that you put some stoppers on couches, and secure down anything else. The shakiness of a shelf or something else may not seem like a bit deal right now, but you never know what the baby will get ahold of, and it is always best to be safe.

## Finish up some projects

If there are some projects that you want to get done around your home, now is the time to work on them. You are not going to have this time once you bring the baby home. So spend some time finishing them up. Whether that includes painting the baby room, cleaning out the cabinets, or you have some other project you and your partner have been discussing, now is the perfect time to work on it. You would be surprised at how quickly time can go after the baby comes and it could be a few years before you get back to them.

## Pack your hospital bags

If you are planning on delivering the baby in the hospital, make sure to pack up a hospital bag ahead of time. You do not want to try to do this while you are in labor and with the bag all ready to go, you can just grab the bag when you are ready to go to the hospital. There are a few things that you can add to the bag. Include some outfits for the baby and some diapers and wipes. Pack some clothes and toiletries for yourself as well since you will most likely spend a few days in the hospital as well. Bring some magazines, a computer, or anything else that you would need to make yourself as comfortable as possible in the hospital.

## Get the car seat

Remember that the hospital is not going to let you take your new baby home until you have a car seat and they are able to see that it is properly installed inside of your car. This can seem like a hassle, but it is meant to keep the baby safe along the way. They will be able to help you learn how to buckle the baby in the car seat and will help you learn how to take the base in and out in case you need to do this before you leave the hospital. Make sure that your car seat is not only safe, that it hasn't gone past its expiration date (you should be able to find this on the bottom of the seat), and that it is installed properly.

# Chapter 2: Getting Through Labor

Probably the one thing that makes new mothers the most nervous about having a baby is getting through labor. They can plan for pretty much anything else that happens, but they worry about the pain, and the whole process, is something that is hard to prepare for. This chapter will discuss some of the most important aspects of going through labor so you can understand what is happening to your body and how you can prepare as much as possible ahead of time.

## Setting up a birth plan

Before you go into labor, it is a good idea to discuss a birthing plan with your doctor or your midwife. This birth plan is just going to be a clear, usually just one-page, statement that will list out your preferences during the birthing process. You should provide a copy of this plan to anyone who will be involved with the birth but do discuss it with your health care provider to make sure they are on board as well.

Work on this plan ahead of time to make sure that you aren't as stressed out about it as you would when waiting until the last minute. There are a lot of things that you can place on this birth plan, but try to keep it simple. You can list out who you would like to be present during the birth, do you want medication, do you want skin to skin contact right after birth, if you will allow fetal monitoring, and so on.

Of course, you do need to make sure that you keep some form of flexibility. Things do happen, and sometimes the doctor will have to make some changes during the delivery of this birthing plan. Having this birth plan can help to answer questions when you are in labor and not in the best position to explain yourself, but having flexibility will ensure that you get the best experience for you and your baby.

## The stages of labor

No matter how much you talk to other mothers or read up on labor, it is truly something that you have to experience to understand what it is about. It is completely different for everyone, and it is really hard to explain what labor is about. But understanding some of the different stages that come with labor will make it easier for most mothers. While we can't get rid of the pain that comes with labor and we can't tell you how long the labor pains are going to last, sometimes knowing exactly what to expect will make all the difference. So let's take a look at the three stages of labor and determine what is going to happen during each one.

### First stage of active labor

To keep things simple, the first stage is going to start when you feel your first contraction and will go until the cervix has had time to dilate to 10 centimeters. It is the longest stage of the birthing process, and a lot of things do happen with it, but it is pretty much going to be the stage until you start pushing that baby out. This first stage is going to start at home, and when it is done, you are within a few minutes of seeing your new bundle of joy. The length of time this first stage of labor is going to vary; some mothers will see it last just a few hours and others will see it last for a day or more.

When this stage starts, you should expect some regular contractions that will last around 30 to 45 seconds. They can feel like really strong menstrual cramps or like a backache depending on what type of labor you are dealing with. In the beginning, the contractions are going to be mild, and they could end up being 30 minutes or so apart. As the labor goes on, the contractions will become a lot closer together and so much stronger.

Many mothers wonder about their water breaking. Some mothers will have the water break early on, and others could be pushing the baby out when the water breaks. It can technically break anytime during your first stage. You should take a note about when it breaks, but this act is not something to worry about because your delivery may be awhile off still.

We are going to assume that your bags are already packed to go to the hospital, so all that you need to do during this stage is to just try to relax. Taking a bath, getting a back rub, listening to music, or even trying to eat can help keep your mind off the contractions a bit. This process is allowing your cervix to open slowly, and you could have a good 12 hours or more of them before you call up the midwife or go to the hospital.

When you start to feel that the contractions are becoming regular and closer together, it is time to keep track of them. When they start to last for about 40 to 60 seconds, and they are four minutes or less apart, going from the start of one contraction to the start of another one, you should make sure that your midwife is on hand or that you head to the doctor. At this point, depending on the mother, you could be somewhere between 4 and 7 cm and the contractions will just get stronger.

If you go to the hospital, they will likely admit you over to a birthing room, and you will be hooked up to monitors to measure the heartbeat of the baby and the strength of the contractions. If you had agreed to get pain medications, this is the time when you will start to get them.

From here, you will probably stay in a pattern for a bit longer. It will probably be similar to one minute of contractions that are pretty strong and then a few minute rest, and it will be on repeat. You can still work with some of your distractions rather than sitting around and feel worried about each contraction. Thinking about things that will keep you calm, doing some deep breathing, and more will really help with this.

This is the part that gets really difficult, and it is important that the people you keep in the room with you are going to be there to keep you calm. You can use pain management drugs if you would like, but some mothers choose to forgo this as well.

As the cervix finishes up to opening to 10 cm, the contractions are going to start being on top of each other. You may hardly get any breaks in between so finding distractions will be hard. The good news is that you are in the final part of it all and soon everything will be over. This intense stage of labor is the final leg of the race, and it rarely lasts more than an hour.

## Stage 2: the big push

For this stage, your cervix has reached 10 cm and is completely dilated. This means that the mother needs to start pushing. You are going to have some contractions, but these are helpful guides to show you when it is time to push. The pain you feel will slowly start to move down your body as the baby is pushed out. The good news is that while pushing can be difficult, it does come naturally. Your body already knows that the baby needs to come out, so it is ready to go.

The amount of time that you take to push will greatly depend on how much medication you get. Those who took epidurals can take up to two hours to push the baby out, but it can be as short as twenty minutes as well. You will need to take quick rests between the pushes so you can be ready for the next stage. You will finally be at the end as soon as the baby crowns.

Once the baby is finally out, your health care provider is going to check the baby's health and will cut the cord. If the baby is healthy, the nurses around you will clean them off, wrap them off, and let you hold your new baby. It is even possible to begin nursing right after the birth too. Some medical centers will even let you hold onto your baby because clamping and cutting the umbilical cord so that you will not have to wait for too long.

## Stage 3: the winding down stage

At this point, your baby is in your arms, and the hard work is done, but there is a little bit more to finish up. You will still need to deliver the placenta. This is usually done within ten minutes, but can sometimes take a bit longer. You will feel a few contractions as the placenta works to separate from the uterine wall, but they are pretty mild compared to what you just went through. The doctor can help finish this by massaging your stomach. You may notice that once the placenta is delivered, you will shake or shiver a bit. Don't worry about this because it is just a natural response to delivery for many new mothers.

If you were not progressing properly with dilating the cervix or your doctor and you discussed it beforehand, you may go with a C-section. This is usually going to require you to spend a few more days in the hospital than before. Vaginal births can usually go home between one to three days, and C-sections will go home within three to five days depending on the complications that may arise. If everything goes smoothly, you get to go home sooner.

# Chapter 3: Those First Few Days at Home

Congratulations! You have given birth to your baby, and now it is time to bring them home. While the pain of labor is now done, there is a whole new set of worries that you need to concentrate on. It is completely natural to be a little concerned about how you and baby will do when you first get home. At the hospital, you had professionals there to help you any time that you needed a break, had a question, or when a concern came up. But at home, it is time to get into your own routine and learn how you and the new baby will start a life together. This chapter is going to give you some tips to help you out during those first few days at home with your newborn.

## Breastfeeding

Many mothers choose to start breastfeeding their babies, and this can start right away in the hospital. Breastfeeding is all natural, provides the best nutrients for your baby, and can be convenient. But this doesn't mean that there are not a few challenges that occur in the process. Some of the tips that you can follow when you are ready to start breastfeeding includes:

- Seek help when needed: mothers who looked for help with breastfeeding were those who saw the most success out of the endeavor.

- Use resources at the hospital: you have a ton of professionals around you in the hospital, why not ask questions while you have them there
- Prepare: keep things on hand for you to do, such as some water and a book to read. Breastfeeding can take some time to be prepared.
- Warm compresses: your breasts can feel sore and sometimes they will become engorged. A heating pad can help with this and can help with the milk flow.

## Sleeping

For the first few weeks, if your baby isn't eating, they are probably asleep. Some newborns will sleep for 16 hours at a time, but remember this is in bursts and not all at once. This can make a new mother really tired and figure out how to deal with the sleep deprivation can be hard. Some of the things that you can do to help with this include:

- Don't obsess over being tired: your main goal right now is to take care of that baby. You will not get the sleep you want so don't even think about it right now.
- Take shifts: you and your partner should take turns with the baby, so you both get a chance to get some sleep.
- Sleep when the baby sleeps: this is a good piece of advice, especially if you don't have

other kids. Both of you can go to bed early or take a nap together.

- Do what works for you: in the first few weeks, don't worry so much about forming habits; those can come later. Let your baby fall asleep on your chest, in the car seat, while rocking or whatever else works.

## Soothing

At some point, you will need to be able to soothe your new baby and make them calm down. In the beginning, you may be unsure about what will help them to stop crying or being fussy. Some of the things that you can try out include:

- Mimic the womb: swinging, holding the baby on their sides, shushing, and swaddling can all mimic how the baby felt in the womb and can make them comfortable.
- Play tunes: something calming, like classical music, can help to keep a baby nice and calm.
- Soak them: a warm bath can sometimes soothe your baby down as well.
- Try something else: each baby will be different, so try something out of the box and see what works.

## Staying sane

You may be super excited to be a new mommy, but all of the cares that your infant requires can be really draining. Finding some ways to take care of yourself, and learning how to lower your expectations a bit so you can steal short breaks can be so important. Some of the things that you can do to stay sane during this stage include:

- Forget the housework: concentrate on just getting to know your new baby. If someone has a complaint, point them to the cleaning supply closet.
- Accept help: if someone is offering, they truly do want to help. Whether it is bringing you a meal, holding the baby so you can take a shower, or something else, let them do it.
- Reconnect: join a mom's group, go to the store, or do something else that will get you out of the house and see other people.
- Pick the bigger jobs: the diaper change really only takes a few minutes. See if those offering to help will take on a bigger job like sweeping the floors, bringing a meal, or even running to the store for you.

## Taking the baby out

If the weather permits it (or you are brave enough to bundle them up and go out anyway), it is a good idea to go out and about with your new baby. Whether it is on a walk, going to visit friends, or making a trip to the store, getting out of the house can be so nice. Some of the ways that you can make this easier includes:

- Enlist some help: take someone you trust with you the first few times you go out. They can help provide you with support and keep you on task.

- Stick to places that like babies: some places are more baby friendly than others. A book store, a library at story hour or some other choice can work nicely.
- Keep the diaper bag ready: there is nothing that is worse than getting your baby all ready to go when you still have to grab your own stuff.
- Keep extra clothes around for you and baby: you just never know when you may need them.
- Embrace the craziness: it is going to be crazy the first few times you go out, so just start to expect this, and things will be easier.

Those first few weeks with a baby are going to be chaotic, and you may be uncertain about what to do at times. But if you take things easy and don't expect things to be perfect, things will work out so much better than you can imagine.

## Taking the baby to their first appointment

If you feel that this is going to be too much for you to handle in the beginning, there is some good news. The first doctor's appointment is going to come up shortly after you bring the baby home, and this is a great place to air your concerns and to ask questions that you may have. For the most part, your pediatrician will want to see the baby within a few days after they head home from the hospital.

At this first visit, the pediatrician is going to perform a physical examination to make sure that the baby is healthy and happy. This will include a height and weight check. You can also ask questions and discuss concerns. Make sure that you are putting your baby in clothing that is pretty easy to take off and bring along a blanket so that it is easier for them to get weighed in the process.

Pediatricians will not only answer the questions that you may have during this appointment, but they will also ask a lot of questions, such as about your home life and the schedule you are starting with the baby. They may want to know how other kids in the family are doing with the baby or they may ask questions to figure out if the mother is tired, run down, depressed, or overly stressed.

It is very important for you to have good communication with your health care provider. This ensures that your baby is getting the best care possible for their situation. Most pediatricians want this open communication, and they are very open to you contacting them with any concerns or questions that you may have, especially during the first year.

One way to prepare for this first visit is to make sure that you have some questions ready. Since you are likely to be very tired from taking care of a baby, put the list in the fridge and add to it any time that a new question comes up. Then you can just grab this list and head out the door whenever you are ready for that first appointment.

# Chapter 4: Tips to Make Breastfeeding Easier

When you bring your baby home, there are two options for feeding your baby. Some people choose to go with formula. They may not want to worry about how breastfeeding will go, or they like the convenience of using the formula so that their partner is able to help with feedings at night. They may even be concerned about going back to work, and they just want to stick with the formula.

Others will choose to breastfeed. While breastfeeding is a great option to go with, it is all natural, has all the nutrients that the baby needs to stay healthy, and it is less expensive than formula, some challenges come with using his option. It is important that new mothers are set up understanding what breastfeeding is all about and the challenges that they may face along the way.

Most people know about all of the benefits that come with breastfeeding. They know that this milk is going to contain all of the nutrients that the baby needs in the right balance. They know that breast milk is easier for the baby to digest compared to commercial formula and that the antibodies are found in breast milk will boost the immune system of the baby. Breastfeeding can even be beneficial to the mother, helping her to lose weight, bond with her baby, and so much more.

Even knowing all of this, some challenges can come with breastfeeding. Your supply may take some time to come in, or you may have trouble making enough to satisfy the baby. Your baby may have trouble latching on or learning how to go with this method. Your breasts may become inflamed or sore from the activity, and it can be really hard to breastfeed when you have to go back to work, and pumping is not that easy or comfortable either.

With all of these concerns, it is no wonder that some new mothers are worried about breastfeeding their newborns. They want to provide their newborns with all of the benefits that come with breast milk, but they are also worried about adding more stress and worries that are already there. If you are considering breastfeeding, here are some of the tips that you can follow to help make this whole process easier.

## Ask for help

Reading online and in books about breastfeeding is a good start, but trying to do it all on your own can be the big challenge. The first time that you breastfeed the baby, which will usually be shortly after delivery if it is possible, make sure to ask for help. There are usually nurses and a lactation consultant available in the hospital who are able to offer tips, such as showing you how to position the baby and to help you learn how to do the latch properly. This is the best place for you to learn because there will be a lot of people around who can help you.

When you get started, you will need to make sure that you are comfortable. You can even support yourself with some pillows if you need. Cradle your baby close to the breast, but do not lean forward and try to bring the breast to the baby or you will be really uncomfortable. Support the head of your baby with one hand and then support your breast with the other one. With your nipple, tickle their lower lip to encourage the baby to open up their mouth wide. The baby will then take in part of the darker area near the nipple, and the nipple should be far back in the baby's mouth. Listen for a swallowing and sucking pattern that is rhythmic from your baby.

If you want to switch the baby around to the other breast, you can release the suction. Don't just pull off though because this can really hurt. Take your finger and gently insert it into the corner of your baby's mouth. This will release the suction so you can move them.

## Let the baby pick the pace

For the first couple of weeks, your baby is going to breastfeed every few hours, day and night. Watch for some of these early signs of hunger to know when it is time to breastfeed. As you start to become familiar with your baby, you will catch on to these signs easier, but look for lip movements, sucking motions, restlessness, and stirring.

Let the baby nurse from the first breast completely, until it starts to feel soft. This will take around fifteen minutes, but remember that there is not really a set time. Some babies will take longer, and some will take shorter. When they seem like they are done with that breast, try to burp them. You can then offer them the second breast. If the baby is hungry after the first breast, they will latch on to the second breast and continue to eat. If they are not hungry, you just need to start the next session on that other breast.

Sometimes the baby will only want to breastfeed on one of your breasts. This is fine, but consider pumping with the other breast to relieve some of the pressure and to make sure that your milk supply stays up.

## Let the baby sleep in your room

For the first few months at least, let the baby sleep in your room. This helps to lower their risk of SIDS, and it can make feedings at night so much easier. Do not let them sleep in your own bed though because they could become trapped and even suffocate on the bed. This can be from the mattress or sheets on the bed or from the parent rolling over on them. Put them in their own bassinette or crib so that they are safe, but still nearby.

## Keep the pacifier away

Some babies will be the happiest when they have something to suck on, even when it is a pacifier. But for some babies, if you give them a pacifier too soon it can interfere with breastfeeding since sucking on this pacifier is going to be different than sucking during breastfeeding.

According to the American Academy of Pediatrics, you should wait until you have established a good breastfeeding routine before you introduce in a pacifier. Pacifiers are not all bad because when a baby sucks on one during bedtime or naptime, it can reduce their risk of SIDS. You just need to make sure to introduce it at the right time, so it doesn't interfere with your breastfeeding efforts.

## Take care of the nipples

In some cases, even if you do everything correctly, your nipples can become sore and uncomfortable. There are a few things that you can do to make this better. After the feedings are done, it is fine to let milk dry on them because this helps to keep the nipples soothed. You can also change out the bra pads in between feedings if you have some leaking because this can get uncomfortable. When you bathe, make sure that you keep the soaps, cleansers, and shampoo down to a minimum because this will irritate the nipples more during breastfeeding.

If your nipples end up becoming cracked or dry, make sure that you use a form of lanolin after each of the feedings. These will help to moisturize your nipples and make them feel better, and it is completely safe for the baby.

## Make good choices

You also have to take care of yourself when it comes to breastfeeding. Everything that you do will affect the breast milk that you are providing to your baby, so you do need to take some precautions. Some of the things that you can do to ensure that you make good lifestyle choices include:

- Eat a healthy diet with lots of nutrients
- Drink lots of water, milk, and juice
- Get as much rest as possible
- Don't smoke
- Be cautious with your medications

Breastfeeding is a great way to provide food and nutrition for your baby and for you both to bond together, but succeeding with breastfeeding can be a challenge. When you learn how to give it some time and follow the other tips in this chapter, you will be able to provide the very best to your baby without quite as much hassle.

# Chapter 5: How to Soothe Your Baby Back to Sleep

As a new parent, you are going to be tired. You want to provide the best for your baby, but you were up going through all the labor and delivery process, and that little bundle of joy is not on a regular schedule of letting you sleep through the night. Dealing with this lack of sleep can be hard for any parent, whether they are with their first child or they are going through this again.

Getting frustrated when your baby won't fall asleep is not the best answer, yet it is so easy for new (and sleep-deprived parents) to feel like things are hopeless. In many cases, this is going to make things worse. The baby will start to feel that you are getting anxious or upset, and that will make things worse. That is why the first step that you need to do anytime that you are trying to soothe your baby back to sleep is to just remain calm. If you can't do this right then (and there will be times when this happens), trade off with your partner for a few minutes to regain yourself.

Once you are sure that you are calm and ready to handle the situation, there are a few other things that you can try out to help soothe your baby down, so they go back to sleep. Some of the tricks that you can try out include;

- Make sure the baby is dry and fed: no baby wants to go to sleep if they are hungry or wet and they are going to cry. This may seem obvious, but when you are sleep-deprived, it is easy to forget these simple things. Make sure to check their diaper and see if they want something to eat and see if this will help.

- Hold the baby: many times, your baby just wants you to hold onto them. You love your baby, and they love you too. They sometimes just want to be comforted, to have their parents hold onto them for a bit. You can't spoil your baby in the first few months, so there is nothing wrong with holding them to help them feel comforted at night.

- Rock the baby: the back and forth movement that you do while rocking can be really comforting to the baby, especially when you are holding the baby. Even a few minutes of this can help your baby calm down.

- Take a walk around the house: sometimes the baby wants a different movement. Something may be bothering them with the rocking, or they want to take in some different scenery. Do a quick walk around the house and see if this is the result that the baby needs.

- Try some music: for some babies, some gentle music is able to ease up the tears a little bit. It can calm them down, distract them a bit, and many babies like to have some soft noise instead of all the silence around them. You can pick out a CD that you like to do this when you aren't in the room or signing works great too.

- Pat or rub their back: as you are holding onto your baby, try to rub their back, either in a circular motion or going up and down. Some babies like to have their back patted. This rhythmic patting can mimic the heartbeat, which is a sound that the baby is very used to so it will be calming to them.

These soothing strategies are pretty simple to work with, and often doing one or two of them will be enough to get the baby to calm down and go back to sleep. You do have to learn what is going to work the best for your baby. Some may like walking around more while others are better with some music or singing. As you become more comfortable with your baby, you will quickly learn what works the best for you.

If you have tried out a few of these options and they are not working, and you are starting to become more frustrated, it is time to take a break. Never get so overworked that you may cause harm to the baby. It is fine to set the baby down in their crib, even if they are still crying, and then walk out of the room for a few minutes to calm down. Yes, they are still crying, but they will be fine while you regain yourself enough to go back into them.

# Chapter 6: The Importance of Self-Care Postpartum

Now that we have taken some time to talk about the ways that you can take care of your newborn once they come home, it is time to talk about how you can take care of yourself a little bit. Many new parents get so involved in taking care of the baby that they forget they need some care as well. While you may be missing out on some of that sleep you are used to at this time, it doesn't mean that you can't work to take care of your body and your mind in other ways. And in reality, if you don't provide some all important self-care to yourself, you are going to start falling behind in the care you provide your newborn. Let's take a look at some of the things that you can do to ensure that you make self-care a priority, even when you are taking care of the baby.

## Making it a priority

The best thing that you can do when you are expecting your new little one is to make sure that you and your partner sit down and go over the expectations that you have for each other. This is the time when you will need to tell your partner that you have to schedule in some self-care time. You may both decide to hire in a housekeeper to come in and clean once a week to help out, you can ask people you know to bring in some meals during those few weeks, or to hire a doula. You can agree that each night the mother gets to go take a bath or go for a walk by herself to clear her head or do something else special.

It doesn't matter what type of plan you come up with, the important part is that it becomes a priority. Waiting until the baby is born is not the best idea because emotions are going to be high and both partners will be low on the sleep they need to think rationally.

## Lower your levels of stress

During that first couple of weeks, you should try to make sure that you are spending some time doing something for yourself each day. It doesn't have to be that complicated or take that long. Something like taking a few moments to drink some coffee, doing some journaling, reading a bit in a new book, or taking a shower. Find something that doesn't take a long time (that you can sneak in during nap time if needed) and will still make you feel good when it is all done.

In addition to doing something small each day, you should find a way to schedule a "mom day" at some point in the first few months. This is something that allows you to get out of the house on your own for a few hours. It can be refreshing to get out without the baby for a little bit, and this special day gives you something to look forward to. Some of the things you can consider doing includes leaving the baby with someone so you can get a nap, getting your hair or nails done, going to pick out a new outfit, read for a few hours in a bookstore, and so much more.

## Get some sleep

As a new mother, you will probably hear all the time that whenever the baby sleeps, you should sleep. This is great advice, but in practice, it doesn't always work out that way. It is hard to fall asleep when the baby is napping. You are probably going to think about all of the things that you could be doing, such as making supper, cleaning the house, and more.

Despite the long to-do list that is running through your head, it is still important to stop and get some sleep. Your body is running on way less sleep than it is used to at this point in the game and this can really mess with your mood and your health. So any time that you are able to sleep, go ahead and do it. When someone comes over, let them hold the baby while you go and take a nap. Let your husband take care of the baby so you can get some sleep. Ignore the dirty dishes and other chores for a bit; no one really cares about these when they come over and if they do, invite them to take over the mess.

Things will get back into the routine that you are used to, and you will get those chores done. But as a new mother, your job right now is to be well rested so you can take care of that baby. So, make sure that you are getting as much sleep as possible.

## Eat right

Yes, this one is going to seem impossible right now. You are already so busy taking care of a newborn and so tired from it all that the only thing you are thinking about is finding food that is fast and doesn't make you spend all day in the kitchen. But it is important to your recovery that you eat healthy foods that are good to the body and to the brain.

Healthy fats need to be a priority in your diet because they are a hormone and brain food. They will help you to feel so much better compared to just grabbing something to eat out all of the time. Remember that one of the biggest risks to postpartum depression is a diet that is poor, so you will need to pick out a diet that will help feed the body in the right way.

This can be hard which is why you should prepare ahead of time. Making some freezer meals to keep on hand for those days when you just can't get to supper can be nice. You can just pull out one of the bags and have dinner ready, with the added bonus of knowing the food is always healthy and yummy for you.

## Get some movement

This does not mean that you need to get right back to your strenuous workout routine that you were doing before you got pregnant. This is actually bad for you. You need to give your body some time to recover after having a baby so take things slow. But sitting around on the couch all day long is not really the answer either.

Getting a little bit of activity each day will help you to feel better in no time. Just put the baby in their stroller and walk around the block a few times a week. Consider finding an easy yoga routine so that you can begin stretching a little bit at a time. The movement will help you to recover more and can increase your mood after having a baby, but you do need to remember to take it slowly during your recovery time.

## Reduce risk of postpartum depression

It is so important to prioritize self-care and rest during those first few weeks after having a baby. If you start out making new habits out of this, it is going to be easier for you to stick with this and get the results that you want, rather than trying to build up a new habit later on.

When you take the time now to take care of yourself, you will find that you are less stressed, will have much lower blood pressure, and you can even have more energy to put towards your new mothering duties. All of these can help you reduce your risk of postpartum mood disorders. If you are not able to give yourself some of the self-care that you need, it is going to be hard to give your baby the care that they need.

Self-care is so important for a new mother who is recovering. This is a part of bringing home a new baby that many new mothers will forget about or put on the back burner, but it is still so important to work with. Take some time for yourself, try to get in some movement (even if it is just a quick walk around the block), let others help you out, and try to eat healthy meals, and you will be amazed at how much easier it is to take care of your newborn.

# Chapter 7: How to Take Care of a Preterm Baby

When a baby is born before they reach the 37th week, they are going to be considered premature and often will be called preemies. This is a new territory, something that you may not have been counting on when you did all of your planning before bringing this new baby home. Most mothers who bring home a preemie baby will b nervous and scared because these babies will have more risks of complications due to being born early.

The complications that could arise are going to increase the earlier that your baby is born. Any of these complications are going to be addressed by professional nurses and doctors in the NICU, or the neonatal intensive care unit. As a new parent, it is important to know what to expect when it comes to taking care of a preterm baby and what your role will be during this time.

Premature babies are not completely ready to deal with life outside of the womb. Their bodies are still going to have some parts that are undeveloped including the immune system, digestive system, skin, and lungs. The part that still needs to develop will often depend on how early the baby was born.

This can sound pretty scary, and you may be worried about how the baby is going to be able to survive outside the womb. The good news is that thanks to medical technology, it is possible for preemies, even those born extremely early, to live until they are strong enough and are developed enough to do all of this on their own.

There are several ways that a preemie will come. Sometimes the body will decide that it is ready to give birth before it is time and the mother is going to feel contractions and the other signs of labor. Often, when the mother gets to the hospital, they will be able to stop the labor and will put her on bed rest in the hopes of keeping the baby in the womb for a bit longer. Sometimes they may not be able to stop the labor, and the baby will be born early.

On the other hand, sometimes the doctor will decide that it is in the best interest of the mother and of the baby to have the baby be born early. There are some conditions, such as elevated blood pressure in the mother, that could make it dangerous for both if the baby stayed in the womb, so it is better for the baby to be born. Your doctor will be able to discuss this with you ahead of time.

Whether your baby is born a few weeks early or a few months early, a premature baby can be a scary experience, and most new parents are not ready to deal with this. The time that the baby is born early will also determine how long they will have to remain under care in the NICU.

The NICU is going to be the new home and protective environment for the baby for a little while. It is a good idea to become familiar with this place so that you know what is going on, who is doing what, and how you should play a role in this area. The NICU is going to have everything that your baby needs to continue developing and to be ready to go home with you including access to physicians in every specialty, respiratory equipment, monitoring systems, and caring staff.

If you have never spent time in the NICU, all of the equipment that is found inside can sometimes seem a bit overwhelming and even scary, especially if this was not a planned thing and you are just out of surgery after giving birth. Learning how all of these machines work will make it easier to relax and will prevent you from getting scared and nervous.

The staff in the NICU will be your best resources to helping you understand these machines and equipment. Each hospital is a bit different, but there is basically going to be every piece of equipment that is needed to help your baby grow big and strong. The staff will spend a lot of time with your baby and you, helping you to understand what is going on and helping to make sure that the baby is developing properly so familiarize yourself with them and don't be afraid to ask them questions if you have these.

**Kangaroo Care**

One type of care that you may be interested in is known as Kangaroo Care. This is a technique where a preemie baby is going to be placed on the mother's bare chest, in an upright position, so that there is tummy to tummy contact between the baby and the mother. The head of the baby will be turned so its ear can be right at the heart of their mothers.

Numerous studies show how this kind of care can greatly help and benefit the baby. Some of the ways that Kangaroo Care can help the preemie baby includes:

- Increased intimacy and bonding: this is so important no matter the baby because it helps them to feel safe.
- Increased weight gain: this kind of care is going to make it easier for your baby to fall into a nice deep sleep, which means that they can take that energy and direct it towards other functions of the body. When the baby increases their weight gain at a faster pace, it means they will stay in the hospital for a shorter amount of time.
- Breastfeeding: this kind of care means that the baby will have easier access to the breast, which will help them to grow. This kind of skin contact will also make it easier for milk production to come in.
- Body temperature: studies have shown that baby's and mothers will have thermal

synchrony. So, if the baby is feeling cold, the mother's body temperature can help to warm them up.

All of this is important to help the baby grow and prosper while in the NICU. Baby needs to have a warmer temperature, the ability to gain weight faster, and even more intimacy so that they feel safe and secure in this new setting. When all of this comes together with the help of Kangaroo Care, it is easier than ever for your baby to get healthier and move out of the NICU faster.

## How can you help?

As a new parent of a preemie baby, you may feel like you are at a loss for what you should do. You want to be there to support your baby and to help them grow, but you may also feel like anything that you do is going to hurt them or won't work the way that you want. While your professional doctor and nursing staff may take over a lot of the medical stuff that your baby needs, it is encouraged for the mother and father to interact as much as possible with the baby.

There are quite a few ways that you are able to interact with your baby and help them to become stronger along the way. Some of the options that you have available include:

- Touch the baby as often as you can. Stroking motions, holding their hands, holding them with Kangaroo Care, or any other option will work really well.
- Talk to the baby. Your baby is already able to recognize your voice, and it is going to be very comforting for them to hear you. You are not just limited to talking to the baby, it is fine to sing or read to the baby.
- Change your baby's diaper, read to them, or do some other regular day things.
- Be there for their first bath. You may have to use sponges or washcloths depending on how your baby is doing.
- Help out with some of the procedures for your baby. This can include simple things such as taking their temperature.

Dealing with the NICU can be a bit scary, and many new parents are not sure how to handle it. The good news is that you can be very involved with the care because this is going to help your baby be ready to go home earlier. Depending on how early the baby was born, it can take them some time to get to come home with you. You can work with your doctor to determine the right milestones that need to be hit so your baby can go home.

# Chapter 8: Bringing Home Multiples

When you find out that you are having twins or more, things are going to be a little bit different. Yes, you will still have some of the same challenges that other mothers have, but now some of those issues are going to be multiplied. For example, just because those two babies look alike doesn't mean that they are going to have the same eating or sleeping schedule.

But the day has finally arrived. You and the multiples are ready to come home. It may have seemed like forever while you were pregnant (that anxiety and worry that comes from carrying multiples can make time drag on), but now it is time to bring them home. Your multiples may already be a few weeks old or more depending on if they needed to stay in the NICU due to their early birth, but the same kind of preparation can be done either way. Take in a deep breath, realize that you may need some more help than other parents and that no matter what, you will be able to adjust to this new life in time.

## First things to consider

When you are bringing home your babies, you need to make sure that you have infant approved car seats. Each state is going to have some different safety standards so make sure that you check on these before purchasing both car seats. You will need one for each baby, and often it is recommended that you purchase them new to make sure that they aren't damaged or compromised in any way. You will need to make sure that these are installed in the car properly. Finding a specialist to help you with this, perhaps before you need to bring the baby home, so you are not under pressure so that you know they are in properly.

## Getting the home ready

You will be able to follow some of the advice that we gave earlier about preparing your home for one baby, but you may have to take some extra considerations and do a little extra work to prepare for two babies. There will be a lot of equipment that you need, but not all of it is needed right away. For example, your babies will not need a high chair right away since they are not able to sit up on their own so you can hold off on this until later.

When picking out some of the supplies that you will use, consider whether you will actually need two of each thing. Many parents of multiples think that because they are having twins or triplets that they need to have that many of each thing. This can get really expensive and is not really necessary. For example, you are probably still fine with just one swing because one baby may rock to sleep in it while the other one is eating or eating on the floor. There are very few times when both babies will want to be in the same contraption at the same time.

Another thing that you will need to have is a place for your babies. You will need to consider whether you want to place them in their own cribs and get them used to that right away or if you want something that will allow them to sleep in your room and is a bit more temporary for now. Doing a twin bassinet can work well to hold the babies in your own room, but at some point, you will want to get them their own cribs as well.

When it comes to picking out a place for the babies to eat, you won't need to work with a high chair right now because they are too little and these chairs are going to take up a lot of space. In the beginning, you may be just fine getting a comfortable chair for yourself for feeding them. Make sure the chair is big enough, so you are able to feed both babies at once if you need.

Keep a lot of the babies' cleaning supplies on hand. This would be things like wipes, diapers, and plenty of changes of clothes. One baby can make a big mess so imagine what two or more are able to do. It is sometimes hard to figure out how many diapers you are going to need ahead of time in each size, so stocking up is a bit of a challenge. If your babies are born early, it is possible that they could stay in the small sizes for a few months. But sometimes these babies can grow fast just like any other baby, and they may need a bigger size a lot sooner than you thought. This means that you will need to keep lots of diapers on hand, but try not to overbuy on them either.

While we are on the subject of diapers, you should consider having a diaper disposal, especially when we are dealing with multiples. You can get a diaper container that contains odor, so your home will still smell good. This is totally optional though because many families will save money on this, and will just throw the diapers into some plastic bags.

## Get some help

When you are bringing home more than one baby at a time, there is going to be a big need for help. It is tough to do this all on your own because you have twice as much work. Your babies will not sleep at the same time or even stay on the same schedule so it can be tough to ever find time for a break for you to get to sleep at night. So before you bring these babies home, it is a good idea to think about the type of help that you want to have.

In most cases, you will be able to find people who are willing to help, and they may already be offering. But it is also important to never be afraid to ask for help when you need it. People want to be there for you, and you are not doing yourself or your babies any favors by trying to do it all on your own. Most of the time people will be thrilled to help you out, so keep a list of those who offer to help and then take them up on that offer whenever you need.

Sometimes, you may need to be direct in what you need for help. Rather than waiting for someone to offer, tell them exactly what you need. If you need an errand done, care for older siblings, pet car, meals prepared, or someone to watch the kids so you can take a nap, make sure to tell others. People are often willing to help, especially when they know your hands are full with multiples, but they may not know what would help you out the most.

**Things to consider:**
As a parent of multiples, there are a few things that you should consider when you bring these new babies home from the hospital. Some of these considerations include:

- You may not be able to bring both babies home at the same time. Sometimes one baby will have more complications than the other after birth, while the other one is ready to go home. This can seem hard, but there are some ways that will make the adjustment easier. If you only need to care for one baby to start with, it will give you a bit of time to catch your breath along the way.
- You do not need to do everything right this second. Some parents get obsessed about childproofing their homes before the babies even get home. But your baby will not be moving all around the home for at least a few months. You do need to do it before they move around, but it doesn't have to be your top priority right now.
- If the babies are born early, or they have other special needs, be aware that there could be some extra medical issues that come up in addition to the normal requirements that come with taking care of an infant. You should work with the caregivers for your babies to

make sure that you learn the proper way to take care of these babies.

- Many times, multiple is going to be born smaller than other babies. This means that some of the outfits you got as gifts or purchased may not fit in the beginning. You may have to rely on preemie clothes, even if they are only born a few weeks early, to help keep them warm.

- Work up to having a schedule. Your babies are not going to be on a good schedule right from birth, and you are working with two, rather than one. You will eventually find a schedule that works for both you and the babies, and it is fine to stick with this one. You can work to get them on the same schedule, but don't worry about whether that schedule makes a lot of sense to other parents.

- Learn how to get to know the babies. Some parents are worried that they will not be able to tell their babies apart, but this is often easier than you can imagine, especially if you take the time to bond and connect with your babies. You will be able to pick up on their personalities and even their cries pretty quickly.

Bringing home multiples can be really challenging for new parents. You may be overwhelmed by what you need to do and how you are going to be able to handle these two different personalities at the same time. But when you learn how to take your time, relax, and provide them with the care and attention that they need, and you will be just fine.

# Chapter 9: Common Concerns with Your Newborn

As a new parent, it is common to have a lot of questions and concerns about how to take care of this baby. Here we are going to take a look at some of the common concerns that parents will have about their newborn and some of the steps that you can take to make sure you get through these hard times.

*How can I encourage my baby to sleep?*

Getting your baby on a sleep schedule can be difficult, and there really isn't a magical way that you can get the baby to fall asleep. But there are a few things that you can try. The first thing to consider is a bedtime ritual for the baby. It isn't reasonable to just expect your baby to fall asleep on their own. Most of the time they will need a bit of a routine to help them out. Playing with them a bit, giving them a bath, getting them warm and comfy, and then rocking them to sleep can really help the baby to relax and fall asleep.

There are a few other things that you can try out as well. You can try to lull them to sleep with a bottle or by breastfeeding, but don't let them fall asleep with this in their mouth to help prevent ear infections and tooth decay. Try out a few different sleeping arrangements to see what is most comfortable for the baby; they may like to sleep in the room with you. And always look to see if there is something that is causing them to have trouble with sleeping, such as being too cold or too hot.

*How can I prevent SIDS?*

Many new parents are worried that they will lose their babies because of SIDS. While it is pretty rare to occur, it is a high worry for most parents. There are a few things that you can do to help prevent SIDS in your baby though, including:

- Provide a healthy environment in the womb: low birth weight and premature birth are two big risks for developing SIDS. Getting good care during pregnancy and eating right will help with this.
- Keep smoking away from the baby: this is considered one of the biggest risk factors for developing SIDS. Make sure that you do not smoke around the baby and keep other smokers away.
- Keep the baby on their back: when the baby is awake, tummy time can help them develop stronger muscles. But at night, the baby needs to sleep on their back.
- Make sure that the environment that you provide the baby to sleep in to help keep SIDS away.

*How can I keep my baby healthy, they seem to get sick often?*

Some babies seem to get sick more often than other children, and this can be hard for a new parent. There are a few things that you can do to help keep your baby healthy and to prevent them from catching every cold and flu that comes along:

Breastfeed as much as possible: babies who get breast milk are less likely to get sick. And even when they do get sick, it is not as severe.

Keep their nose clear: if the baby's nose gets clogged, get some nasal drops and use a nasal aspirator to help clean them out. This helps to keep the infections out.

Keep your home and the sleeping environment clean: when their sleeping environment is clean, it is easier for the baby to stay healthy.

Take them to their doctor visits: this is the best way to make sure your baby stays healthy. It will ensure that your baby gets the immunizations that they need to stay healthy.

*When should I discipline by child*

When you have a baby, it is not really about disciplining your baby, although you are starting to build the bonds of trust and showing your baby the right way to behave. For example, when you childproof your home, you are setting limits on where the baby is allowed to play. When you say no, you are helping the baby learn when they are headed for trouble. You should not discipline your child really at this time, just concentrate on getting some of the right boundaries.

*How will I be able to balance a job and parenting*

Many parents choose to work outside of the home after their baby is born, but this can cause a lot of tension and worry for a new parent. They want to still be there and form those attachments to their baby, but they still need to leave home to earn an income. The good news is that there are a few things that you can do to make sure you keep those close bonds, even when you have to head back to work:

- Share the work: if both of the spouses in your home have to work, it is important that both parents will take on some household chores so that they can both spend time with the baby as well.
- Happy departure and reunion: before you head off to work, cuddle the baby and make them feel good, and then do the same thing once you come home. If you are breastfeeding, let the caregiver know that they should not feed the baby right before you get home so that you can use this as your bonding time.
- Attachment time: when you are with the baby, it is fine to use attachment time. You can use a baby carrier when you are cleaning or doing errands so that you and the baby get plenty of time together.

*How do I get my spouse to help out more?*

You thought you were getting into this together, but now it seems like you are the only one who is doing all of the work. This can make it hard for a tired mom to take on all of the work. Sometimes it is simply because your spouse needs to be taught how and when to help out. The first thing that you can do is to choose the tasks that you need a lot of help with and then do them with your partner. Pont out the techniques that work for you, but let them have a chance to try out things on their own.

You should also consider letting dad be home all alone with the baby at times. You will be surprised in most cases about how well dad can do on their own. If you are breastfeeding, make sure to feed the baby before you go or leave some milk behind to help him out. And then when dad is dealing with the crying baby, don't just come to the rescue all of the time. Let them have some time to work it out on their own sometimes.

*Is my baby getting enough nutrition?*

It is hard to tell sometimes whether your baby is getting the right amount of nutrition to stay healthy. This is why it is helpful to go to the doctor when required because they are able to track the baby's weight and will tell you. Then after a few months, you will be better able to tell if the baby stays healthy or not.

Let's take a look at the breastfed infant. By the time the baby is a week old, a well-fed baby who is breastfeeding will have about six wet diapers a day with a few stools. If you feel that the milk is letting down, and you hear the sucking and swallowing noises, it is likely that your baby is going to be getting plenty of nutrition. It is pretty normal for a baby to lose some weight when they are born, but they will gain it back pretty quickly if they are getting the right nutrition. You can visit with your pediatrician to determine if the baby is getting the right nutrition along the way.

It is sometimes easier to tell if the bottle-fed infant is getting the right amount of nutrition. As a newborn, they only going to take about two ounces at each feeding, but by the first month, they may be up to four ounces. A good rule of thumb is that your baby will take in about two ounces of formula each day for each pound they weigh. So if your baby is 10 pounds, they will probably take in about 20 to 30 ounces each day.

# Conclusion

Thanks for making it through to the end of this book, let's hope it was informative and able to provide you with all of the tools you need to achieve your goals whatever they may be.

The next step is to start following some of the tips that are in this guidebook. Some of these are going to be pretty easy to implement, and you can even get started on a few, such as preparing your home, before the baby is even born. As a new parent, you are sure to have a lot of questions and concerns, and this guidebook is going to help you learn how to take care of your baby and yourself, without feeling too overwhelmed.

This guidebook is the guide that all new parents need to read to help them prepare before their baby arrives. We will talk about how to prepare your home, how to get ready for labor, how to get through those first few days of having the baby home including how to help them sleep and how to breastfeed, and even how to take care of yourself. There are also sections about how to take care of a preemie baby and what to do when you bring home multiples.

When you are expecting a new baby, and you want to make sure that you are as prepared as possible, make sure to read through this guidebook to learn everything that you need.

Finally, if you found this book useful in any way, a review on Amazon is always appreciated!

77178546R00071

Made in the USA
San Bernardino, CA
20 May 2018